Blockchain Applications in Healthcare

Dr. Tanupriya Choudhury would like to dedicate this book to The Indian Army for their dedication, sacrifice and excellency towards our motherland India and he would also love to dedicate this book to his parents Sri Mrigendra Choudhury and Smt. Minakshi Choudhury, his beloved wife Rituparna Choudhury and beloved son Rajrup Choudhury for their immense support throughout this work. He would also like to dedicate this book to his research guides Prof. (Dr.) Vivek Kumar, Prof. (Dr.) V Cyril Raj, Prof. Sumathy Eswaran and Dr. Darshika Nigam, who have always mentored him during his master's and doctoral research.

Mr. Abhirup Khanna would like to dedicate this book to his parents Mr. Ravi Khanna and Mrs. Abha Khanna for all their blessings, love and support. Mr. Abhirup Khanna would also like to dedicate this book to Dr. Sapna Jain, Dr. Anushree Sah and Dr. Divya Srivastava for their warmth, compassion and esteemed council.

Mr. Abhishek Bhattacharya would like to dedicate this book to his family.

Prof. (Dr.) Jung-Sup Um would like to dedicate this book to his family and workplace.

Dr. Prasenjit Chatterjee would like to dedicate this book to his grandparents, his father late Dipak Kumar Chatterjee, his mother Mrs. Kalyani Chatterjee, his beloved wife Amrita and his little angel Aheli.

International Perspectives in Decision Analytics and Operations Research Set

coordinated by
Prasenjit Chatterjee

Volume 1

Blockchain Applications in Healthcare

Innovations and Practices

Tanupriya Choudhury
Abhirup Khanna
Prasenjit Chatterjee
Jung-Sup Um
Abhishek Bhattacharya

iSTE

WILEY

First published 2023 in Great Britain and the United States by ISTE Ltd and John Wiley & Sons, Inc.

ISTE Ltd
27-37 St George's Road
London SW19 4EU
UK

www.iste.co.uk

John Wiley & Sons, Inc.
111 River Street
Hoboken, NJ 07030
USA

www.wiley.com

Library of Congress Control Number: 2022948726

British Library Cataloguing-in-Publication Data
A CIP record for this book is available from the British Library
ISBN 978-1-78630-894-8

Contents

Foreword

Due to the vast amount of health-related data, Blockchain technology offers a significant answer in applications related to healthcare. With the help of a peer-to-peer network, Blockchain technology records each cryptocurrency transaction. The fundamental goal of Blockchain is to provide high-end security in order to address the problems that arise in handling healthcare data more effectively. Many scholars have focused their efforts on this subject with the goal of providing extensive research on the introduction to Blockchain, its platforms and different consensus algorithms. The movement of its uses towards healthcare and medical-related data has also attracted the attention of researchers. Aside from mentioning Blockchain technology, the writers have also mentioned the use of the IoT (Internet of Things) and AI (Artificial Intelligence), which together define the next technological era. The editors have done an excellent job of combining a number of chapters from autonomic computing with the viewpoint of applications connected to healthcare. The editors have also done a good job of providing a thorough review of the application of Blockchain technology in healthcare. The book helps readers become more knowledgeable about how Blockchain technology is being used in healthcare-related applications, such as maintaining patient monitoring systems. In order to combine the benefits of both technologies, it also elaborates on how Blockchain and the IoT may work together. We strongly believe that the book explores Blockchain and healthcare researchers.

Dr. Praveen KUMAR
Associate Professor
Amity University, Tashkent, Uzbekistan

Dr. Roohi SILLE
Assistant Professor
University of Petroleum and Energy Studies (UPES)
Dehradun, Uttarakhand, India

Preface

The healthcare sector has always been an important part of society. With the recent outbreak of a pandemic, the importance of a robust, efficient, secure and patient-centric healthcare industry has never been more apparent. Blockchain is a new technology that keeps a record of every transaction performed using a cryptocurrency across server computers that are linked in a peer-to-peer network. Blockchain enables transactions to be secure, transparent and reliable. The question of revolutionizing the healthcare sector is being seen across various countries across the world and Blockchain could be integral in achieving this goal. The applicability of Blockchain in the healthcare domain can be seen as a remarkable opportunity by researchers and scientists across the globe for solving pertinent real-world problems dealing with patient records, medical supply chains, wearable diagnostic tools and telemedicine sessions. This book focuses on the fundamentals of Blockchain technology along with the means and methods of its integration with the healthcare industry. It provides an exploration of the current challenges in the healthcare sector and how Blockchain technology can provide solutions to these issues. It dives deep into specific areas where Blockchain technology can be adopted in the healthcare industry, such as patient data privacy protection, pharmaceutical supply chain, clinical trials and genomics. This book serves as a resource for readers to understand the fundamentals of Blockchain and the IoT (Internet of Things) across various application areas of healthcare and identify futuristic problem areas resulting from technological convergence. It also talks through futuristic research areas for the healthcare industry wherein Blockchain and its allied technologies can prove beneficial. However, it is important to note that these are only potential benefits and no guarantees can be made about their effectiveness. This book has a total of 11 chapters.

Chapter 1 proposes a framework for managing and operating a healthcare system using Blockchain technology. The framework aims to present a detailed overview of all the actors in a healthcare ecosystem, their working principles and ways of communication. Moreover, the authors present a comprehensive integration of other technologies such as the IoT and machine learning with the proposed framework.

Chapter 2 deals with the concept of smart contracts. It discusses the role of smart contracts in ensuring seamless transactions among various intermediaries. This chapter illustrates the creation and working of smart contracts along with their set of benefits. Furthermore, we discuss specific use cases involving the implementation of smart contacts for streamlining complex processes.

Chapter 3 discusses various platforms for the implementation of Blockchain technology. This chapter aims to present a detailed analysis of prominent Blockchain platforms such as Ethereum, Hyperledger Fabric, Multichain, etc.

Chapter 4 looks at the variety of challenges faced while implementing techniques from Blockchain technology in healthcare. This may include data protection and data sharing challenges, cross-border information sharing challenges, data security challenges, challenges in stakeholder management using an appropriate permissioned network, and study challenges.

Chapter 5 discusses growing concerns about medical data security in an online ecosystem. This chapter explores present-day data ownership laws and compliance regulations dealing with the administration of medical records. It illustrates the means and methods of creating an interoperable decentralized Blockchain-enabled health record system. Moreover, the authors illustrate the problem faced by many in terms of the number of devices used in a healthcare system and the manageability of the vast variety of data generated.

Chapter 6 presents the proposed system that connects with methods such as on-chain and off-chain communication patterns to allow patients and healthcare professionals to share personal health records. This chapter proposes a scheme that emphasizes the importance of maintaining a true fair-exchange policy when transferring medical records without the involvement of a trusted third party.

Chapter 7 explores ways in which Blockchain can assist in preventing access and misuse of patient data by third part intermediates. The authors illustrate the means of strict and efficient implementation of data privacy laws by the use of smart contracts and consensus algorithms. Identification of data controllers and perspectives on anonymity and pseudonymity are discussed in later parts of the chapter.

Chapter 8 describes a Blockchain-enabled fragmented personal fitness facts ecosystem that enables unique drug discovery, biomarker development and preventative healthcare procedures, as well as secure personal records using

Blockchain and deep learning technologies to connect users and providers of personal records with medical records.

Chapter 9 discusses the life-cycles of software development through the component-based software engineering approach. Furthermore, we discuss how to create a Blockchain-based repository that stores software components and also discuss how Blockchain technology helps to secure our data in healthcare applications. The proposed software development life-cycle model ensures the security of user data and also improves the quality of healthcare applications.

Chapter 10 discusses the role of smart contracts and Blockchain technology in healthcare and other use cases. Smart contracts are computer protocols that facilitate, verify or enforce the negotiation or performance of a contract. Smart contracts were first proposed by Nick Szabo in 1996. He defined a smart contract as "a set of promises, specified in digital form, including protocols within which the parties perform on these promises". Since then, much research has been conducted on smart contracts and their potential applications. Some challenges that have been identified include scalability issues and the need for more user-friendly interfaces. Despite these challenges, many companies are already using smart contracts in various ways. For example, some companies use them to create digital wallets or to streamline supply chain management processes.

Chapter 11 describes the future aspects of Blockchain and the healthcare industry. Blockchain technology has the potential to revolutionize healthcare research by providing a secure, decentralized platform for storing and sharing data. This could potentially allow for more efficient and accurate clinical trials, as well as better tracking of patient outcomes. While there are still some challenges to be overcome, such as ensuring data quality and privacy, the future potential of Blockchain in healthcare is very exciting. These points will be discussed throughout this chapter.

We hope that our efforts are appreciated and the reader benefits from this book.

Tanupriya CHOUDHURY
Abhirup KHANNA
Prasenjit CHATTERJEE
Jung-Sup UM
Abhishek BHATTACHARYA
November 2022

Acknowledgments

Dr. Tanupriya Choudhury and Mr. Abhirup Khanna would like to thank their work place, the University of Petroleum and Energy Studies, Dehradun, India for creating a positive research environment to start this proposal. They would like to thank all the contributors from different countries and especially the reviewers throughout the globe who helped review the chapters to improve the quality of the book. They are also thankful to the senior leadership of UPES and the administration for giving them the opportunity to work on BAHIP 2022 and providing them with all possible support. They are thankful to Sh. Sharad Mehra, CEO, GUS-Asia for his "all-time-go-ahead" blessings and freedom of work. The Honorable Vice-Chancellor Dr. Sunil Rai has continuously supported us as a torchbearer, big thanks to you sir for your mentorship. They would like to thank everyone for their involvement and willingness to take on the completion of tasks beyond their comfort zone. See you all in the next edition of the book. We also acknowledge the support of Dr. Roohi Sille during the editing of the chapters at the final stage of publication.

Mr. Abhishek Bhattacharya would like to thank his family for all their support.

Dr. Jung-Sup Um is grateful to his workplace, Kyungpook National University, South Korea, for supporting and providing him with such a working environment that he could devote time to such projects.

Dr. Prasenjit Chatterjee wishes to thank his family for all their support.

1

Framework for Blockchain in Healthcare

Blockchain technology could be seen as one of the uptakes from the field of digitization that has attracted the attention of researchers and academicians over recent years. A Blockchain is a distributed database with an immutable committed block that provides transparency and robustness, which are the inherent characteristics of the architecture of Blockchain. Blockchain can also be understood as the set of connections which are interconnected to provide the connection in the entire architecture. Blockchain has been recognized as a development for addressing the distribution issues of information with the significant characterization towards data privacy and information security. Thus, the focus here has been to highlight the state of art in terms of Blockchain development, personalization, applications and limitations within the healthcare sector.

Blockchain is one of the most innovative and crucial advancements in the technology world. It belongs to the professional world, bringing together the distributed ledger technology with its architecture and applications in the medical field. This framework will include the evolution and ownership aspects of Blockchain along with the working principles and the different methods in the healthcare ecosystem. Since Blockchain is one of the technologies which is being used in the improvement of the prevailing standards of data sharing, handling and security, the growing anticipation of Blockchain, with its data management ranging from the traditional to its extensions, will be discussed. Emphasizing the benefits of Blockchain in healthcare, this chapter will also go over the challenges and limitations of Blockchain. The present editorial will also make efforts to approach the challenges of Blockchain in healthcare. A comprehensive interpretability in Blockchain with its open issues and future trends will be described. This

Chapter written by Neha MEHTA, Jyoti AHLAWAT and Leena ARYA.

enhancement in the medical field has also set the path of a new revolution in transforming the individual sectors in the healthcare industry. Thus, the focus has been on showing the direction of persistent revolution towards the potential of Blockchain technology in making efforts to establish innovation in the healthcare industry.

1.1. Concept of Blockchain

A Blockchain is a system for storing data in a manner so that it becomes impossible or extremely difficult to hack or change the system. Blockchain is generally a book of digital transactions, which are first copied and circulated across the complete network of systems present in the Blockchain architecture. All the blocks present in the chain are made up of a number of complete transactions, including each time any new transaction occurs for the system of Blockchain, a newly entered transaction is entered into each participant's book. And whenever there are multiple participants, the multiple participant architecture is managed by the decentralized database, which is popularly called distributed ledger technology (DLT). *Blockchain* may be marked as a common and permanent book that organizes the activity of record keeping in a network of blocks through input transactions, new insertions and asset tracking. According to Ahram et al. (2017), Blockchain presents a safer way for exchanging service and information transactions.

An asset might be physical (e.g. a car) or intangible (e.g. land), physical (patient treatment) or intellectual (creative property, patents, copyrights, branding) data or medical records (personal information, laboratory results, medical findings, history of diseases, doctor's prescription). Things of value can be followed virtually and can also be alternated on a network of Blockchain, via cost cutting, along with the reduced risk for all those users involved in it. Blockchain is a DLT in which all the transactions are documented through an enduring cryptographic signature known as a hash.

Blockchain has provided a platform that can improve the transparency as well as authenticity of healthcare data, maintaining permissions and also streamlining the claim process (Angraal et al. 2017).

Blockchain is a form of dashed information. The quicker it is received, the more accuracy it preserves. Blockchain provides each shared piece of data and all of the entirely transparent data that is stored on an accounting book immediately, but only the network's members that have permission have access to it. Hence, according to the researchers, Blockchain is considered to be an ideal way for delivering information, although Blockchain has always faced the limiting issues of latency and throughput, solutions to which have been given by many researchers such as ECBC produced by Xu et al. (2017). A Blockchain can track prescriptions, records, clinical data, payments, medication, a patient's accounts much more, where people can believe that every single piece data is true, and the user can see all the details of the transactions to give greater confidence, end-to-end communication, new efficiencies and greater opportunities. But, due to the newly developed technology, it still has a very limited number of users (Aru 2017), along with certain challenges and limitations towards the development of Blockchain applications, including security, scalability, speed, privacy, interoperability and patient management (Agbo et al. 2018).

How does Blockchain initiate?

Blockchain rests on three major concepts: **the Blocks, the Miners and the Nodes.**

The Blocks

Every Blockchain consists of various numbers of blocks, along with the three primary elements in each block, which are:

– **data**: acting as an input for the block;

– **nonce**: a 32-bit entity based number referred to as a **nonce.** When any block is created, the nonce is generated randomly which further achieves a "hash" as a block header;

– **hash:** a 256-bit number and linked to the nonce, which appears with a large number of 0s.

A nonce develops the cryptographic hash, whenever the initial (first) block of a Blockchain emerges. Then, the acknowledgement is done for unless it is dug, the data in the block is signed and connected to the nonce and hash.

The Miners' association

The newly developed blocks in the chain are generated through a development procedure known as mining. Every block in the Blockchain mining of a block is not evident, especially for the larger chains, because each block has its unique nonce and hash, as well as the hash of the previous block in the chain. Miners are special pieces of software that solve the strangely complex math nonce finding problem that generates an accepted hash. Because the hash is 256 bits and the nonce is only 32 bits, there are approximately four billion nonce–hash possible combinations that need to be mined after finding the right one. This block is then added to the chain, which when it appears is referred to by the miners as the "golden nonce".

All of the blocks that come after changing the previously existing block in the chain necessitate re-mining; hence, it is always reported as a tough job to manipulate Blockchain technology. Thus, as a "safety in math", finding golden nonces needs a long time and much computer power. This modification must be approved by all existing devices in the system, and if a block is successfully mined, the miner is compensated financially.

Nodes

Nodes are any type of electronic device that helps in keeping the network functioning and in maintaining the copies of the Blockchain. Any newly introduced mined block for the Blockchain needs to be verified, trusted and also updated for each node with its own copy of the Blockchain, and the network must also be algorithmically approved. Each action performed in the ledger is easily checked and viewed due to the transparent nature of the Blockchains, where each member is identified with a different alphanumeric identification number, showing their transactions.

The Blockchain also maintains its integrity and develops trust among its users, thus combining public information with a reliable scalability of trust and a system of checks-and-balances through efficient use of technology.

Components of basic Blockchain

Distributed ledger technology (DLT) is used by all network participants which are involved in the Blockchain and have an access to the distributed book and its maintenance of the record of transactions. The shared ledger allows the transactions to be recorded only once, and any duplicate efforts to be discarded, as has always been found in typical classical networks. The different attributes of the distributed ledger technology are presented in Figure 1.1.

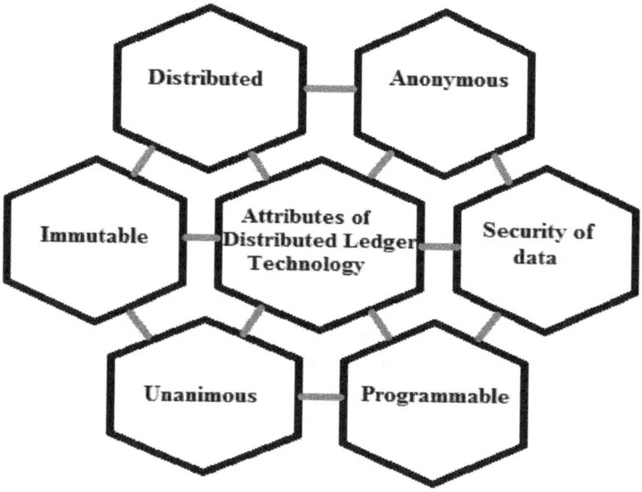

Figure 1.1. *The attributes of distributed ledger technology*

Immutable records

In Blockchain technology, none of the members are allowed to change the input after a transaction has been recorded in the common ledger, nor can they modify or tamper with it. However, it does give the following opportunity: if a transaction record contains an error, then a new transaction will need to be combined in order to reverse the error; then both the transactions will be cleared.

Contracts that are smart

Smart contracts are a collection of rules for completing transactions quickly, which is gathered on the Blockchain for its automatic execution. A smart contract describes conditions and regulations for incorporating, combining terms for the data, guaranteed services and much more.

Benefits of Blockchain

Operations generally squander time and money on duplicate records and third-party verification. The recorded systems may also be liable to cyber attacks and fraud; therefore, the defined data verification can be slowed by transparency. Transaction volumes have exploded as a result of the Internet of Things (IoT). As a result, every process takes longer towards the end result drains – or necessitates a better move, namely, entry into the Blockchain.

As a member of a members-only system, we can be sure that we are getting correct and timely data, because the classified Blockchain documents will only be shared with network members to whom access is given. According to Dey et al. (2017), all network members must agree to data efficiency, and then all verified transactions are fixed as they are always stored. A transaction cannot be deleted by anyone, not even a system authority. The time-consuming record agreements are often rejected with a vanished ledger that is shared across network participants. A set of rules to speed up the transactions, known as a smart contract, are executed automatically and can be stored on the Blockchain. For example, one of the most well known (and maybe most controversial) applications of Blockchain are cryptocurrencies, like Bitcoin, Ethereum or Litecoin, which can be used to buy goods and services. Cryptocurrencies are digital currencies (or tokens). Crypto can be used to buy everything from your lunch to your next home just like a digital form of cash. Online transactions are always recorded and secured so, despite the currency, cryptography employs Blockchain to serve as a public ledger as well as a data encryption system. Researchers have also given examples of using Blockchains for energy transactions, as in Park et al. (2018).

As far as healthcare is concerned, the devices related to the IoT use the real-time data of the patient, which is processed and further analyzed. Thus, Blockchain in accommodation with the IoT is one of the reasonable choices for e-healthcare systems (Ray et al. 2020).

Blockchain networks

A Blockchain network might be public, private, federated or developed by consortia, among other options.

Blockchain networks open to the public

A public Blockchain, like Bitcoin, is one that anybody may register and contribute to. The disadvantages of a public Blockchain include no or little transaction privacy, inadequate security and a high processing power requirement.

Network of private Blockchains

A private Blockchain resembles a distributed mentoring or public Blockchain network in appearance. However, if one entity manages the network, implements a shared ledger, maintains the public database and controls who is allowed to participate based on the utilization case, trust and confidence amongst participants will skyrocket. A Blockchain frequently runs under a company's security and might be handled on-site.

Blockchain networks with permissions

Businesses that discover a specific chain will often discover a highly secure Blockchain network. It is vital to note that public Blockchain networks can also be described as being of a restrictive nature where one is allowed to join the network and specific transactions. Participants must get either an involved participation or hitch permission.

Blockchain in a consortium

Multiple entities can share the burden of maintaining Blockchain architecture. This is before the entities decide who has access to the information and who is allowed to make transactions. When all players must have permission and share responsibility for the Blockchain, a consortium Blockchain is the way to go. In this category, significant processing power is necessary, but only a small amount of it is available.

1.2. Blockchain as distributed database

Even though the terms bitcoin and Blockchain technology (DLT) are often used interchangeably, they are not interchangeable. To allow Blockchain technology, bitcoin employs a variety of technologies, including distributed ledger technology. Digital signatures, distributed (peer-to-peer) networking and encoding techniques are the additional technologies and computational/mathematical techniques used in Blockchain technology to link the recordings (block) of a database. Blockchain technology might be classified as a distributed ledger.

A Blockchain is a decentralized and permanent ledger that may be used to take possession, transact data, evaluate the effectiveness and assure visibility, safety, confidence and currency transfers in a range of electronic asset transactions.

Distributed ledger technology is based on Blockchain technology across a distributed database that serves as a ledger and an encoded database that stores transaction records. DLT is a cutting-edge database solution with such a knowledge base in which encryption is used in each transactional update and confirmation is feasible across the particular public Blockchain, based on the platform's aim and shareholders. Blockchain technology has progressed from a buzzword to a reality.

Despite being hyped at the present, Blockchain is just one of a list of solutions that are incredibly relevant within the context of, among other things, the transition to digital (but for many applications being from the early phases of hype cycles). It is not the panacea for all problems (far from it), because as the hype goes, it is also quite useful in selected situations whereby the use is appropriate. (Multiple) Blockchain technologies are being used and tested in a range of digital trust and exchanging use situations in industry, in and across cryptocurrency, and also as a contract basis to provide faith in the digital world. Over the next few years, DLT is expected to be among the fastest developing digitalization developments, with a vital role in numerous relevant application cases inside the digitalization of multiple methods and industry.

The hype around cryptocurrency also creates a huge gap between what a technology could conceivably achieve and what it actually can do. Furthermore, there is no denying that distributed ledger technology is gaining traction in the commercial world, particularly in the financial sector. There will be various reasons that DLT adoption is predicted to accelerate throughout all use cases and industry, though in many cases it will fall short of expectations or be unnecessary.

Business projects advancing Blockchain technology

Many corporations, both world leaders and leadership in their particular nations or regions throughout numerous sectors, launched key bitcoin and DLT efforts in 2017 or 2018. Simply looking at the clients of a few key efforts, we can note projects, such as IBM's cross-border transaction bitcoin action plan, that also primarily will have industries from the Asian region on board. This was how it started and it was then confirmed in October 2017 to still be on the verge of reaching 100 industries. At the same time, most of these projects will fall short of their goals, whereas others will grow in importance. Therefore, while various use cases and initiatives as produced by the researchers have been investigated more profoundly, DLT has been introduced to businesses. For a variety of reasons, Blockchain technology is very new, especially outside the scope of bitcoin and cryptocurrencies, which would be the domain beyond which most commercial projects desire of using DLT.

According to Zhou et al. (2020), the Blockchain also has a wide application for the health record management system, where the system uses Blockchain as a storage tool. One of the most prominent issues facing the modern-day clinical system is data handling, which in turn has drastically hampered the efficiency of the medical systems and their process of further development. Moreover, the data breaches that occur to this day are just one of the regular tasks that are committed for the theft of medical data in a similar way to the theft of banking data. Certain projects have been started, including the medical chain. The goal of this project was to develop a single version of the patient's data and thus give them the ability to share their data with anybody in their network. The medical chain unites pharmacy research, therapeutic, operational, prescribed and insurance data through the Blockchain-based application, myclinic.com. Medibloc is another Blockchain-based healthcare project that works on the structuring of big data. Medibloc delivers its service from an application called Medipass. Another, most promising Blockchain-based project in 2020, Dentacoin, has combined the dental industry with the Blockchain industry. The application has accommodated about 2,000 dentists along with 100 locations in a single board. After its launch in 2017, Dentacoin provided many platforms, leading to further improvements. DentaVox is also one of the applications that has served for collecting information and conducting research surveys. Dentacare is another application that provides education aids related to dental care. Another is Robomed Network; this project has been created to help the healthcare ecosystem thrive and thus gives a universal care solution. The Robomed Network has produced a different range of EMR/CRM solutions.

1.3. Architecture of Blockchain in healthcare

Blockchain as a ledger technology has a continuous list of transactions and data records. It simplifies and expedites healthcare and its related processes. The interoperability nature along with the property of supply chain validation allows us to dramatically reduce the back office load, data management and maintenance cost. There are five key areas in healthcare that are promptly driven by Blockchain technology.

1) Online access – the Blockchain allows patients to have online access to their longitudinal medical records, providing them with the security key and thus allowing the interoperability of data.

2) Maintenance of health records – the Blockchain allows the longitudinal way of maintaining healthcare records. It also maintains a secure medical record between multiple healthcare organizations and the patient. This gives the futuristic approach to the Blockchain.

3) Automation of adjudication of health claims – the smart architecture of Blockchain allows the execution of the transactions of the contract, which helps the support of compliance audits as well as the completion of a claim through the business rules. Thus, it also follows the concept of disintermediation.

4) Management of supply chain – using a supply chain, we may improve the efficiency of your business. The Blockchain enables contract healthcare through real-time health tracking and execution. This architectural feature of Blockchain management also benefits the contract administration and thus reduces its costs. This

approach also innervates the satisfied and completed contracts that provide the consumers with information about quality and sources of the facilities (including drugs) being provided.

5) Interoperable nature – this feature of the Blockchain enhances the efficiency of the Blockchain by facilitating and encapsulating the large amount of patient data, thus providing further health initiatives. It promotes the additional high transaction in volume of patient data, along with the negotiation of chain data with the consortium of the views of healthcare experts. The Blockchain architecture, shown in Figure 1.2, consists of two main blocks, the transaction block and the maintenance block. The transaction block, which consists of several blocks through different network sources, tends to transmit the data towards the Blockchain in different time slots. Each time a new transaction occurs, it is transmitted to the network of computers which are connected worldwide. The network then checks and confirms the validity of the transaction that has occurred and thus allows it to become clustered within the block. All of these blocks are then chained with each other, and the entire transaction is said to be completed.

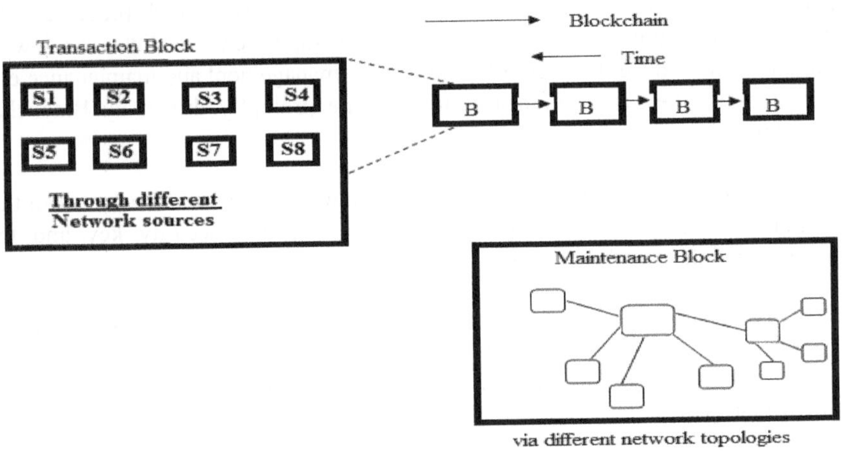

Figure 1.2. *Blockchain architecture*

Figure 1.3 shows the schematic of data blocks.

The Blockchain architecture is a decentralized type of P to P architecture, where the different digital transactions are recorded in the distributed network within the shared ledger. These digital transactions are the copy of encrypted signal data which are structured in the block format with the index pointing towards the earlier block. Where the members stored the copy of the shared ledger and these changes made in the shared ledger are reflected to all. All the original data of original size as a stream towards the data make the implementation of Blockchain in healthcare, as given in Figure 1.4.

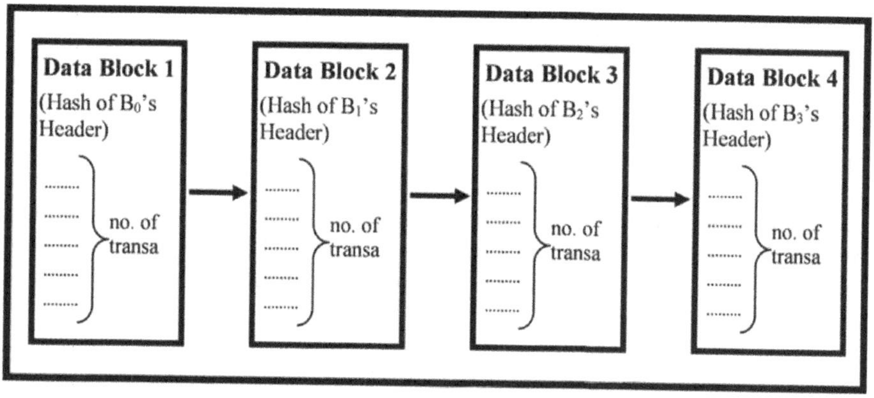

Figure 1.3. *Schematic of data blocks*

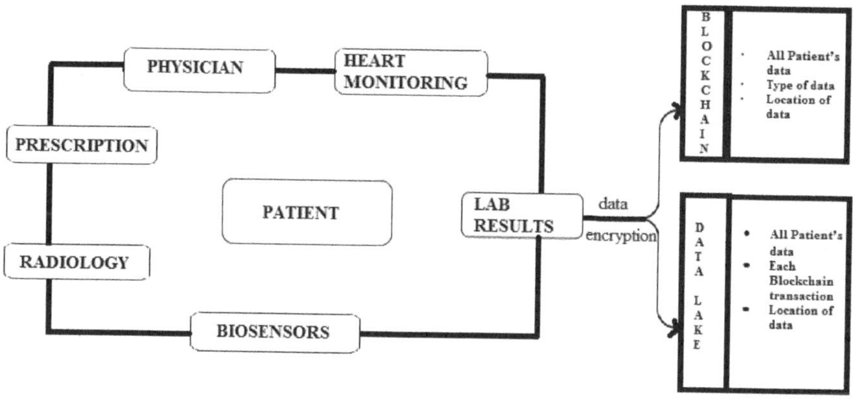

Figure 1.4. *The Blockchain implementation in healthcare*

The Blockchain is the shared and distributed infrastructure that addresses the interoperability and thus provides a comprehensive view of the health data along with the healthcare entities. In this way, the Blockchain offers an efficient approach towards the interoperability and establishes the architecture for health IT, where the patient is encompassed within a chain having completed several activities like prescription, monitoring, radiology, laboratory and biosensors, whichever is applicable to them and the data encrypted is in the form of blocks leading its path towards the Blockchain and the data lake. Each time the data is entered, a new block is accomplished in the ledger and it also acts as an entry in the data lake.

Due to its large architecture and its wide usage of technologies, the patient data remains inaccessible; thus, many studies have confronted this shortcoming of the Blockchain along with its security constraint. Thus, studies have addressed the security concern (Dagher et al. 2018), along with the designing of information management systems, like Medlock (Fan et al. 2018), for handling the patient data. A separate domain related to Blockchain in healthcare has also come into effect through the application of Blockchain in the pharmaceutical industry, as produced by Haq and Esuka (2018), where a permissioned Blockchain is applied to track the movement of drugs from manufacturing up to its delivery and thus recording its after-effects.

1.4. Development of Blockchain: A state of art

The Blockchain is a distributed chain of blocks that keeps track of all transactions across several computers around the world, prevents its alteration and, after that, is recorded in such a manner that Blockchain improves data security (Kuo et al. 2017) while also making data interchange more cost-effective and public. It also assigns third parties for whom the primary function is to provide a certificate aspect between transactions and trust (like as in banks and notaries).

Many researchers have discussed the importance of cryptocurrencies, which has piqued the interest for businesses in various industries, with banking becoming one of the most prominent at the moment. With digital payment apps through healthcare apps, there is something for everyone and thousands of new job positions, and Blockchain has appeared in such a way towards the development of new enterprises.

The extensive knowledge of the technical team for cryptocurrencies, either as prototypes or even a manufacturing system, virtualized computation and data analytics helps to take advantage of the benefits of Blockchain, and thus to figure out the best Blockchains for Ethereum, Tezos, Hyperledger, EOS, NEO and Qtum among the projects and the liability for when to employ private permission Blockchain technology like Quorum. A few capabilities and possibilities with Blockchains are figured out as follows:

– with web3, solidity, cakeshop and truffles can launch and develop Blockchain applications among the engineering capabilities;

– OpenZeppelin and smart contracts are two examples of bespoke dapp frameworks;

– Python is used for application and data science engineering;

– Swift and Objective-C are used to create enterprise native mobile apps;

– Phoneix/Elixir-based web applications with serverless architecture;

– case studies on the Blockchain technology;

– infrastructure for the Blockchain;

– Blockchain and mobile banking;

– Blockchain and peer-to-peer transfers;

– Blockchain and digital money;

– markets and Blockchain;

– marketplaces and Blockchain;

– healthcare and Blockchain;

– application on the Blockchain;

– e-government and Blockchain;

– Blockchain and the banking industry;

– financial technology (fintech) applications;

– regulatory frameworks and Blockchain;

– adoption of Blockchain is hampered by a number of obstacles;

– contracts that are smart;

– Blockchain technology is advancing;

– Blockchain provides privacy, security and identity.

Blockchain has swiftly gained notoriety because of its ability to establish a massive, worldwide shared ledger ability to record everything of value, which was originally created as part of the technology that underpins Bitcoin. A Blockchain is a digital, public distributed log that keeps precise replicas from each of the channel's users' computers. New entries can be made by any party, and prior entries can be reviewed.

In a Blockchain, activities are recorded and transmitted one after another (hence it is named as "Blockchain"). Because previous transactions cannot be erased or falsified, encryption protects the linkages among blocks and its contents. This implies that there is no central body or mediator in the transaction network and ledger. Blockchain technology's ability to instantly store, preserve and circulate every form or asset in a decentralized, automated manner has grabbed the curiosity of entrepreneurs and also the financial services sector as a whole, who really anticipate possible uses and application in a variety of fields. The efficiency of Blockchain and its nevertheless practical effects are evaluated by researchers through various empirical investigations as in Risius et al. (2017) and have justified the multidisciplinary approach of Blockchain.

Blockchain in markets

Blockchain technology has the potential to streamline and simplify the entire market procedure, as well as to create a business assets life-cycle where all entities involved in the transaction have access to the information. Within that situation, a system will save a lot of money on infrastructures, increase transparency, speed up processing cycles, enable easy access to data or even eliminate certain intermediaries like dealers. Nasdaq was one of the first financial service companies to develop a Blockchain-enabled product. Private firms use Nasdaq Linq to handle their company's shares, and it leverages cryptocurrencies – power capitalization table.

Blockchain for performing cross-border activities

Blockchain has the potential to enhance pass transactions through accelerating and deaccelerating the process, cutting expenses and removing unnecessary steps, several of the traditional intermediaries. At the same time, it may reduce the cost of money remittances. Until now, remittance costs have ranged from 5 to 20%. Blockchain is a technology making it possible to cut prices by 2 percentage points to 3 percentage points of the entire value and to provide secured, actual cross-border payments. Using a smart phone app to make real-time foreign payments in the United Kingdom, Santander was the very first firm to embrace Blockchain technology. The solution, which makes use of Ripple's technology, is the creation of a bitcoin Ripple payment system and exchange network. Blockchain is also being used to improve digital identification, where the users are able to select how they represent themselves or with whom their identification is disclosed after their identity online is shifted to a Blockchain-enabled infrastructure and thus can still register their identities on a Blockchain; however, when they require it, customers do not need to re-register with each network operator, as long as those suppliers also are connected to the Blockchain.

This Blockchain application is frequently used as an illustration of understanding requirements in which a digitized single source of identifiable details could allow more frictionless bank accounts, reduced resources and expenses, while retaining privacy.

1.5. Information distribution in Blockchain

For the analysis of data distribution and accountability with the rise of the IoT and 5G, an increasing amount of critical data are being gathered, particularly for the electric management system, whose general steady operation depends on the security of data sharing and transmission. Firdaus et al. (2018) have investigated the security issues along with their solutions like the inter-planetary system (Dey et al. 2017) for privacy in data transfer architecture for smart wearable services in order to provide a balance of performance and resource optimization. Researchers proposed an associated cctv data protection system as well as a private protecting video encoding and storing technology.

Every user in the proposed model has the ability to communicate and receive data from others. The information is not immediately communicated between users (e.g. A and B), but rather through the following three processes:

1) Sensitive data is initially encoded and saved in IPFS via user A. Everybody can receive the encoded material based on a hash function, and only the person who possesses the keys may read it.

2) If A wishes to send data to B, they create a record in the Blockchain indicating that data D has been sent to B. The document also includes an access to data D that is encoded by a distributed chain of blocks that keeps track of B's public key, allowing only B to get the key and retrieve information D to A.

3) The compound annual is used to ensure that the information transfer records are non-repudiable. To improve the system, a practical Byzantine fault tolerance (PBFT) compound annual is adopted. Unlike the commonly used PoW or PoS consensus protocols, PBFT can operate without the need for a token or money, which is also not required inside the electrical data management situation.

1.6. The growing anticipation of Blockchain

The Blockchain is an immutable ledger and is shared by peers, with records of transactions that are always appended in a successive manner. The distributed decentralization is more beneficial to be implemented in healthcare applications, as it is free from the centralized authority. Both concepts of distributed ledger technology and Blockchain are frequently used interchangeably. The overall type of technology is distributed ledger, and Blockchain is a specific form with more technical details. Both inquire about the concept of a ledger, which is a file that records who owns what. According to the research findings in Dey et al. (2017), there are four key characteristics of a distributed ledger: i) payment data that is shared by network members, ii) consensus-based updates, iii) time-stamped records with cryptographic signatures and iv) a vandal enforceable record with all transactions. Blockchain gives the ability to update database entries in a sequential manner using chained cryptography hash-linked blocks (every step performs a hash of the previous block, thus joining transaction blocks through an unbreakable string, hence the term "Blockchain"). The two forms of Blockchains are public and private Blockchains.

Blockchains that are open to the public, can be used by anyone such as Bitcoin and Ethereum, and no one knows who they are. Private Blockchains, which are used by governments and industry consortiums, are similar to a corporate intranet in that users are known and credentialed. One of the most crucial motivations of adopting ICT may be cyber security. Recent data breaches – the Equifax credit scandal where an estimated 145.5 million Americans' personal information was exposed as a result of the incident and also the identities, email and passcodes of 2.5 billion Yahoo user profiles were stolen – highlight the immediate necessity improved security measures. Blockchain systems are a tempting target for thieves, but decentralized store records backed with cryptographic signatures over Blockchain technology could significantly increase network security. Decentralized solutions are supposed to provide increased user control and permissioning of private data. Distributed ledgers are referred to as "trustless" because they do away with the need to rely on any third institution, such as Equifax or Yahoo, inside the midst of private information exchanges. Blockchains are smart networks with no third-party intermediates that can authenticate and transmit value. A sophisticated protocol that identifies, verifies, confirms and distributes transactions inside the network incorporates intelligence straight into the network's processes.

In the healthcare domain, the immutability property that does not allow the Blockchain users to alter or modify any of the records is already appended to the Blockchain. The Blockchain ensures the validity as well as the integrity of the patient records. However, the smart contracts, which are also supported by the Blockchain, are the rules that controls the flow of the patient's record. According to European rules, the GDPR (General Data Protection Regulation) refuses to process any personal or sensitive data of any patient unless there is explicit consent. Thus, as per the growing anticipation, the Blockchain can be associated with the development of an EMR-based clinical management system in compliance with GDPR. As a result, a trust-free system emerges in which human counterparts and organizations do not need to be known or authorized. Rather, the computationally intelligent network is trusted, which could aid in the development of the next digital solutions.

1.6.1. *Challenges faced by Blockchain*

The Blockchain in healthcare serves for multiple issues including data security, care regularity issues, coordination and interoperability, since this industry has a variety of data inputs on a regular basis such as medical records, test results, prescriptions and much more. Thus, the potential benefits are as follows.

Scalability

The first and most important issue is adoption and scalability. Although the transaction network is able to process hundreds of transactions per second without fail, there might be an unusual lag in processing.

Interoperability

The second major issue that must be solved is interoperability, which is frequently cited as one of the main reasons why it is yet to implement the technologies. Because they are unable to send and receive data from some other Blockchain-based systems, many Blockchains create silos and do not interact with other peer groups.

To address this, a number of projects have been established to address the issue. For example, the Smart Bridges design is used to bridge the communication gap between Ark's networks. The technology aims to provide worldwide compatibility and global communication and transmission.

Consumption of energy

The solid evidence technique is used by the technology to verify transactions and ensure that they are trustworthy enough to be added to a system. This technique necessitates a substantial amount of computer power in order to solve complicated mathematical riddles, process, validate and more importantly, protect the entire system.

To solve this problem, Ethereum's co-founder came up with the solution of changing proof-of-work to proof-of-stake. Participants do not have to answer complex puzzles when this approach is used, which saves gobs of energy.

Talent deficit

The requirement of experts is growing steadily, yet finding high-quality people is typically considered as a significant obstacle when considering the digital technology deployment.

Many corporate executives, organizations and policymakers can undoubtedly benefit from this technology. Nonetheless, there are a few setbacks that are contributing to the technology's sluggish acceptance. Similarly, as of 2019, the global market for cryptocurrency developers has increased by more than 517% over the previous year. Despite its enormous gains, the majority of people regard Bitcoin as just a field known. Despite the increased demand for Blockchain developers, there is a severe shortage.

Is standardization still lacking?

This is just a question that has yet to be answered: What standardization does Blockchain adhere to? Despite the numerous networks which exist, there really is no uniform standard. Because of a lack of standardization, concerns like compatibility, increased prices and complicated procedures arise, rendering widespread adoption unfeasible. Due to the lack of a standard version of Blockchain technology, it is going to act as just an obstacle to new companies and users. Aside from the issues listed above, the opposing problems for large-scale deployments are expenses, privacy terms and security issues.

1.7. The benefits of Blockchain in healthcare

The Blockchain benefits healthcare in five different ways.

1) Managing the patient records in longitudinal way

The management of patient records through regular compiling medical records, disease registries, laboratory findings, inpatient ambulatory data and treatments through Blockchain. The wearable data providers are also arising multiple improved approaches to provide care.

2) Indexes of master patients

When working with healthcare data, records are frequently mismatched or duplicated. Also, every different EHR is prepared with a different schema for each field and thus there arise alternative ways of entering and manipulating only knowledge sets. But in Blockchain processing, the full data set, not just the initial key, is encrypted to a logbook.

The user can search for different addresses as there are numerous locations and keys available, resulting in a single patient identity.

3) Adjudication of claims

Because Blockchain operates on a confirmation interchange, all statements are easily known, and the contract is then implemented after the network has agreed. Since there is no centralized entity in the Blockchain design, there is a lower risk of mistakes or cheating.

4) Management of the supply chain

The design of Blockchain-based contracts can benefit healthcare businesses by tracking supply–demand cycles through supply chain management. The entire management includes monitoring how the transaction is happening, checking for the success of the contract and reporting if any transactions or delays are incorrect.

5) Connectivity

Connectivity is a pledge by the chain, which is frequently realized using complex APIs to create EHR compatibility and secure data storage.

The Blockchain networks, which are shared with approved service providers in a safe and standardized manner, are well known for removing the burden of data reconciliation from Blockchains. Other complex activities addressed by the Blockchain, namely through interoperability, include medicine supply management, fraud eradication, clinical studies or revenue cycle management transformation.

1.8. Open issues related to Blockchain

There are varieties of issues related to Blockchain associated with its applications. Some of these are mentioned below.

Blockchain is incorporated with an environmental expenditure

Encryption is the mechanism that Blockchain uses to provide security and get consensus from a distributed network. The actual meaning is just to demonstrate if a person has the power to write down just onto the chains intricate procedures which should be executed, each of which will require a massive amount of processing power. After all, of course, it comes with a cost. Using the most widely used cryptocurrency as an example, it was estimated that last year the computing expected to maintain the running system used the same amount of energy as that of 159 countries.

Hence, it requires sophisticated and computationally costly protection. Smaller Blockchain technologies that are mostly used privately by a corporation to record and maintain commercial activity will use a portion of those sophisticated

Blockchains. Nonetheless, this is a significant aspect, as are the natural ramifications, because energy prices cannot be overlooked.

A dangerous environment is created by a lack of regulation

An unregulated environment is usually a big stumbling block for the value-based ledger systems due to the increasing risk of data hacking at various levels of processing. That may be due to the larger number of networks available, highly unstable market scenarios or due to the lack of government oversight, scams and market manipulation. There is always the risk that perhaps the swap or Internet block in which the user maintains their tokens/valuable information would be subject to hacking attempts, closed down by government bodies attributable to deceptive dealings, as well as disappear entirely. Furthermore, this really is typically the result of a global absence of government regulation. The benefits are difficult for end-users to comprehend due to their complexity.

Although the anticipated revolutionary applications of Blockchain are easy and safer to implement along with the concepts like encrypted and shared ledgering, it requires a lot of time and learning before the "person in the street" will realize how Blockchain technologies are always so useful.

It is no surprise the first Blockchain technology, cryptocurrency, rose to prominence in the aftermath of the 2008 economic trouble, when the media and public opinion expressed broad unhappiness and rising suspicion of existing financial institutions and instruments. Is there really a desire to demolish savings programs and reconstruct them from the ground up 10 years later, with no immediate threat of a repeat? Who knows what is going to happen next? Of course, the past recession was mostly unanticipated, and world events may fuel the need for changes, yet till they do, Blockchain may be a difficult sell for just a number of people.

Blockchains can indeed be sluggish or inconvenient to use

Blockchain transactions (Zhou et al. 2020) could be processed quickly because of their intricacy and encryption and flexible architecture, especially compared to "conventional" methods that can take many hours, showing that the concept has faults. In general, the approach could be used for Blockchain networks that are used for purposes other than storing data, such as inside interactions in an IoT setting, documenting payments and many more. Even as computer access and publishing to a network grows, these chains – which are essentially simply computer files – may become bulky and complex. Ideally, this is really a problem that could be remedied with developments in engineering and computing speed.

Therefore, it is believed that, although these difficulties may offer substantial challenges, Blockchain technology would certainly develop in the near future. And besides, technical progress, like the natural world, has a method of navigating itself its own across intentionally erected hurdles.

1.9. Future trends of Blockchain

Blockchain technology is approaching the stage of maturity with the great enhancement of new start-ups. Furthermore, the Blockchain could also guarantee integrity and non-modification of the entered medical record, which in turn may have repercussions both for keeping track of the outcomes and better documentation of medical errors. However, the tracking of the outcomes in the pharma supply chain also aims to guarantee the integrity of the medicines and other pharmaceutical products. The creation and updation of the directories of healthcare providers is also the support-receiving field of the Blockchain. However, working for the energy requirements of the Blockchain is also one of the prime concerns nowadays along with favorable speed and scalability.

The major themes for future trends of Blockchain include consent management. In the consent management task, the patient consents to data exchange, treatments and privacy preferences are marked to bring in a further improvement in the industry in order to secure and improve the healthcare data management by moving towards the precision of healthcare outcomes.

1.10. References

Agbo, C.C., Mahmoud, Q.H., Eklund, J.M. (2018). Blockchain technology in healthcare: A systematic review. *MDPI Journal, Healthcare*, 7(56), 1–30.

Ahram, T., Sargolzaei, A., Sargolzaei, S., Daniels, J., Amaba, B. (2017). Blockchain technology innovations. *2017 IEEE Technology & Engineering Management Conference (TEMSCON)*, doi: 10.1109/TEMSCON.2017.7998367.

Angraal, S., Krumholz, H.M., Schulz, W.L. (2017). Blockchain technology: Applications in health care. *Circulation: Cardiovascular Quality and Outcomes*, 10(9), e003800.

Aru, I. (2017). Full stack development tools lowering Blockchain entry. *Cointelegraph* [Online]. Available at: https://cointelegraph.com/news/full-stack-development-tools-lowering-blockchain-entry-barriers.

Dagher, G.G., Mohler, J., Milojkovic, M., Marella, P.B. (2018). Ancile: Privacy-preserving framework for access control and interoperability of electronic health records using blockchain technology. *Sustainable Cities and Society*, 39(1), 283–297.

Dey, T., Jaiswal, S., Sunderkrishnan, S., Katre, N. (2017). A medical use case of Internet of Things and Blockchain. *Proceedings of the 2017 International Conference on Intelligent Sustainable Systems (ICISS)*, Palladam, India.

Fan, K.,Wang, S., Ren, Y., Li, H., Yang, Y. (2018). Medblock: Efficient and secure medical data sharing via blockchain. *Journal of Medical Systems*, 42(8), 136.

Firdaus, A., Anuar, N.B., Ab Razak, M.F., Hashem, I.A.T., Bachok, S., Sangaiah, A.K. (2018). Root exploit detection and features optimization: Mobile device and Blockchain based medical data management. *Journal of Medical Systems*, 42, 112.

Haq, I. and Esuka, O.M. (2018). Blockchain technology in pharmaceutical industry to prevent counterfeit drugs. *International Journal of Computer Applications*, 180(25), 8–12.

Kuo Ting, T., Kim, H.E., Machado, L.O. (2017). Blockchain distributed ledger technologies for biomedical and healthcare applications. *Journal of the American Medical Informatics Association*, 24(6), 1211–1220.

Park, L.W., Lee, S., Chang, H. (2018). A sustainable home energy prosumer-chain methodology with energy tags over the blockchain. *Sustainability, MDPI*, 10(3), 658.

Ray, P.P., Dash, D., Salah, K., Kumar, N. (2020). Blockchain for IoT-based healthcare: Background, consensus, platforms, and use cases. *IEEE System Journal*, 99, 1–10.

Risius, M. and Spohrer, K. (2017). A blockchain research framework. *Business & Information Systems Engineering*, 59(6), 385–409.

Wong, M.C., Yee, K.C., Nøhr, C. (2018). Socio-technical considerations for the use of Blockchain technology in healthcare. *Studies in Health Technology and Informatics*, 247, 636–640.

Xu, Y., Zhao, S., Kong, L., Zheng, Y., Zhang, S., Li, Q. (2017). ECBC: A high performance educational certificate blockchain with efficient query. In *Theoretical Aspects of Computing – ICTAC 2017*, D. Van Hung and D. Kapur (eds). Springer, Cham.

Zhou, L., Wang, L., Sun, Y. (2020). MIStore: A Blockchain-based medical insurance storage system. *Journal of Medical Systems*, 42(8), 149.

2

Role of Smart Contracts in Blockchain

Blockchain offers several advantages, including decentralization, persistence, anonymity and auditability. Cryptocurrency, banking sectors, risk assessment, the Internet of Things (IoT) and individual and public services are all examples of Blockchain applications. Because of the rapid expansion of cryptocurrencies, as well as its fundamental Blockchain technology, frameworks such as Hyperledger and Ethereum have emerged to enable a wide range of smart contracts. Smart contracts are computational systems designed to digitally ease, validate or control the implementation of new contracts. Smart contracts have a variety of applications in different domains, including investment banking economic models and the IoT, among others. This chapter covers the introduction to Blockchain technology along with its characteristics and types. It provides detailed information about smart contracts, their working, platforms, programming languages and application areas. It also covers the applications of Blockchain technology in different domains and concludes with the challenges in implementing smart contracts.

2.1. Introduction to Blockchain

Recently, cryptocurrency has piqued the interest of both practitioners and academicians. Bitcoin is generally referred to as the original cryptocurrency. With the capital market surpassing $10 billion in 2016, accomplishment has been achieved (CoinDesk 2016a). The Blockchain is Bitcoin's central mechanism. Blockchain technology was initially suggested in 2008 and was deployed in 2009 (Bitcoin n.d.).

Blockchain is similar to a distributed ledger, for all completed events recorded in a chain of blocks. As more blocks enter the system, it continues to grow. Decentralization, persistence, anonymity and auditability are important properties of

---

Chapter written by Avita KATAL, Teoh Teik TOE and Tanupriya CHOUDHURY.

Blockchain technology. Blockchain may operate in a decentralized environment by combining many basic technologies such as cryptographic hashing, digital signatures and a distributed consensus process. As a result, Blockchain has the potential to significantly reduce costs while also increasing efficiency. Furthermore, as the quantity of provider user information and vulnerable devices rises, the deployment of secure, reliable and verified services is critical. Unfortunately, trust is becoming increasingly rare as the amount of information thefts at monolithic technology companies rises, exposing huge amounts of private data. Centralization, a fundamental flaw in many software architectures, provides an uneven relationship among users and suppliers, making the personalized security of electronic information impossible while offering a single point of failure for hackers to attack.

Blockchain is a decentralized, irreversible transaction ledger in which every transaction is inextricably linked to the one before it. Working in untrusted distributed environments may well be safeguarded by both the ledger of information and distributed agreement on the authenticity of the transaction, as the Blockchain technology's fundamental purpose. Furthermore, transactions incorporate operational code, allowing software services to be provided between untrusted users. Since it was initially used in cryptocurrencies, interest in Blockchain technology has grown in both industry and academia, as they assess the applicability and functioning of the underlying Blockchain technologies.

To enable Blockchain decentralization, nodes involved in transactions and block generation should be able to verify the validity of new updated blocks to the chain. In this scenario, the nodes should reach a consensus since there is no trustworthy centralized method to make such a judgment. Various consensus techniques have been used to achieve such an accord (Katal et al. 2021). These versions must all work towards the same goal: identifying whether transactions inside the Blockchain are legitimate by verifying the activity of each new block introduced to the chain. The differences are in who can add blocks and at what rate, as well as the issue used to reach agreement. Consensus is commonly used to describe "mining", or the solution of a complicated problem that is easily verifiable but difficult to overturn.

The method by which a miner contributes additional blocks to the network is known as mining. Each block in a chain has its own distinct nonce and hash, and connects to the hash of a block before it is in the network, making the mining of a block challenging, particularly in big chains. Miners use sophisticated programs to tackle the extremely difficult mathematics problem of creating a valid hash. Making changes to any prior block in the chain involves re-mining not only the altered block, but also all following blocks. Hence, it is so difficult to manipulate Blockchains. Consider it "math safety", because finding golden nonces requires a considerable amount of effort and computational power. Whenever a block is properly processed, the alteration is accepted by all nodes in the system and the miner is rewarded economically. Figure 2.1 shows the working of Blockchain technology.

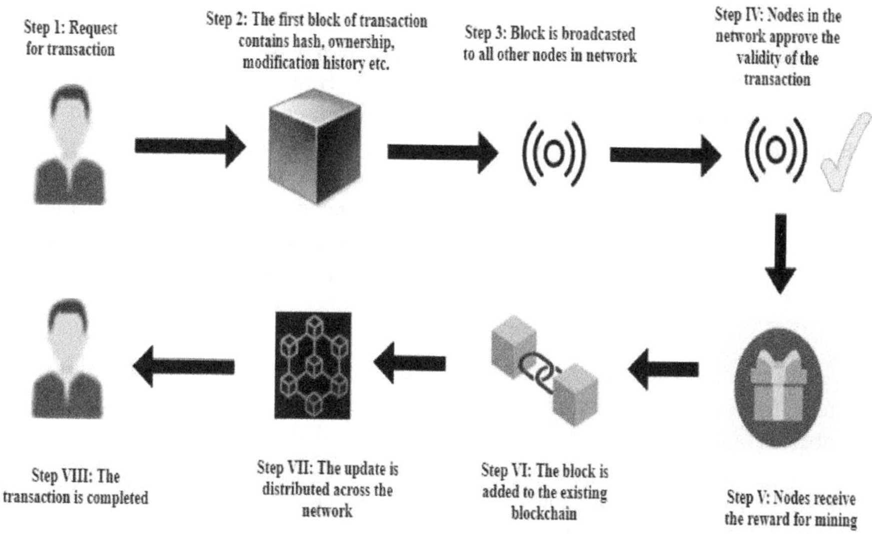

Figure 2.1. *Working of Blockchain. For a color version this figure, see www.iste.co.uk/choudhury/blockchain.zip*

2.1.1. *Types of Blockchain*

Public Blockchain: Anyone with Internet connectivity may use Blockchain technology in the public Blockchain (Idelberger et al. 2016). Everyone has access to the transaction details and the verification of the same. Members of the public Blockchain may engage throughout the consensus protocol. Bitcoin and Ethereum are two mechanisms that make use of public Blockchain technology.

– Hybrid Blockchain: a hybrid Blockchain's information is either private or public. There are hybrid Blockchain systems that are partially decentralized. A Hyperledger is one of the major examples of approaches that employ hybrid Blockchain systems.

– Private Blockchain: the write privileges of the blocks in a private Blockchain are managed by a specific authority, whilst the read permission is either public or limited. The range of nodes that can join this Blockchain is restricted (Pilkington 2016). The Blockchain's transaction information is not accessible to every node. This Blockchain is extremely safe.

2.1.2. *Characteristics of Blockchain*

– Decentralization: each operation in typical centralized transaction processing systems should be verified by a trusted centralized agency (e.g. the central bank). A Blockchain transaction can be performed between any two identities (P2P) without verification by a central authority. As a result, Blockchain has the potential to significantly reduce hosting expenditures (both planning and production costs), while also eliminating compatibility issues in the centralized computer.

– Persistence: since each transaction propagated over the network must be validated and stored in blocks dispersed across the entire system, every transmitted transaction will also be validated by many other peers and checked. As a result, any fabrication may be quickly recognized.

– Anonymity: a created address may be used by any entity to join the Blockchain system. Moreover, to avoid disclosing their identity, a person may create a huge number of addresses. There is no longer a centralized entity that safeguards the confidential information of the user. This method ensures a certain level of anonymity for the Blockchain's transactions. It should be noted that Blockchain cannot ensure complete anonymity.

– Auditability: since each transaction on the Blockchain is verified and timestamped, users can easily track and audit prior records by connecting to the node in the decentralized system. Each operation in the Blockchain network may be monitored back to prior transactions repeatedly. It optimizes the transparency and traceability of Blockchain-stored data.

2.2. Smart contracts

Nick Szabo proposed that a range of contractual requirements may be encoded in software and hardware to make contract violations expensive (Wang et al. 2019). A smart contract (SC), according to Nick Szabo, is an electronic protocol used for transaction that carries out the conditions of the contract. The main advantage of having smart contracts above commercial procurement is the speed of the control layer; for example, adopting smart contracts makes it much easier to keep records of contractual partners' prior behavior. Contract words can include references to legal contracts and are self-enforcing. Smart contracts reduce the danger of deliberate and unintentional exceptions, as well as the need for trusted intermediates. An intelligent agent is a smart contract. In other terms, it is a computer software that can make choices if specific criteria are satisfied. An agent's intelligence is determined by the intricacy of the transaction it is designed to complete. Contracts can be extremely simple transactions completed in seconds or minutes, or they can be very complicated and protracted transactions, including talks and tens of pages of written language with particular rights and duties that may take hours or months to accomplish. Smart contracts are currently classified as relatively basic transactions. All descriptions in (CoinDesk 2016b) were divided into two main types by the author: smart legal contracts and SC code. SC code is defined as "code that is validated, stored and implemented on a block-chain" (CoinDesk 2016b). The functioning of an SC is entirely reliant on the coding language that is used to show the agreement and the Blockchain's capabilities. The term "smart legal contract" refers to code that may be used to supplement or replace legal contracts. The functionality of this SC is determined by legal, political and business institutions, rather than technology. A balance, secure storage and program code are all features of a smart contract. The contract condition is made up of the storage and balance. When the contract is fulfilled, the information is saved and changed on the Blockchain. Each contract is given a distinct 20-byte address. The contract code cannot be modified once it has been posted on the Blockchain. A contract may be executed by simply submitting a transaction to the contract's address. This operation is performed by each agreement node (also known as miners) on the system in order to attain an agreement on its conclusion. The status of the contract will be revised as necessary. It can comprehend its personal storage, put funds into its account, deliver orders or payment via user profile deals and even build new contracts depending on the activity it gets.

2.2.1. *Operating mechanism of smart contracts*

SCs are made up of a collection of rules of procedure and logic called scenario response logic. In other terms, they are distributed, reliable shared programs implemented on Blockchain. The participants entering a contract must decide on contract agreements, leakage in contract terms, breach of contract obligations and outside validation information sources (oracles), and place it on the system as a smart contract to execute contract implementation on their own.

Figure 2.2 depicts the smart contract working mechanism. Even after participants have accepted the smart contracts, these are frequently linked to the Blockchain in the type of machine code.

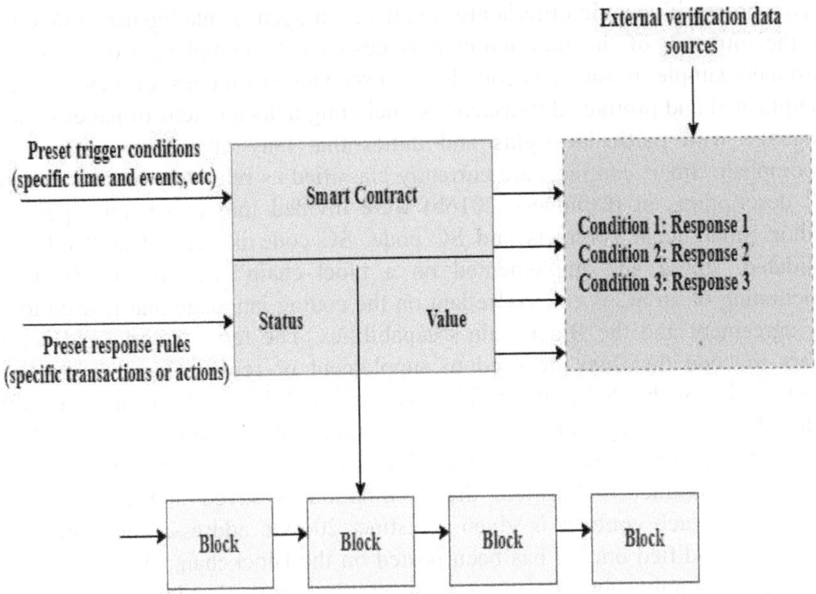

Figure 2.2. *Operating mechanisms of a smart contract. For a color version this figure, see www.iste.co.uk/choudhury/blockchain.zip*

2.2.2. *Applications of smart contracts*

2.2.2.1. *Finance*

Smart contracts and Blockchain enhance transparency and trust among players, while reducing infrastructure, transaction and administrative expenses. The following are a few examples of smart contract applications in finance (Ojetunde et al. 2019).

– Security: the security sector entails complicated operations that are time consuming, wasteful, inconvenient and risky. Smart contracts can avoid the use of middlemen in the securities custody chain. The centralized clearance process necessitates time-consuming operations, as well as complicated external and internal reconciliation.

– Insurance: every year, the insurance industry invests millions of dollars in claim processing while losing millions to fraudulent claims. They could be used to automate insurance claims, validation and payment, boosting claim processing speed while reducing fraud and minimizing potential risks (Gatteschi et al. 2018).

– Trade finance: currently, trade finance is riddled with inefficiencies, and the business is particularly prone to theft. Furthermore, the trading procedures on the basis of paper finance must be modernized or supplanted with digitized activities. They enable organizations to autonomously initiate commercial activities based on pre-set criteria, increasing productivity by simplifying procedures and lowering fraud and compliance expenses.

2.2.2.2. *Management (Lutz Maicher et al. 2016)*

Smart contracts provided by Blockchain can give adequate accountability for management roles, duties and decision-making procedures. The following are some examples of use cases.

– Management of digital properties and rights: Maicher et al. (2016) argued for the use of smart contracts to authenticate intellectual property existence and authorship. Smart contracts may also be used to control digital rights. For example, once a musician's work is used commercially, a dApp called Ujo Music enforces royalty payments (ConsenSys Mesh n.d.).

– Organizational management: most businesses are now governed and focused on a board of directors who make the bulk of decisions. The future of organizational administration is expected to be flattened and decentralized. Smart contracts can eliminate the need for intermediaries that impose false constraints and overly complicated laws.

– E-Government: smart contracts can help to increase the efficiency and authority of the E-Government by simplifying bureaucratic processes. Other smart contract applications include innovative payment methods for labor and pensions, E-Voting (Ayed 2017; McCorry et al. 2017) and so on.

2.2.2.3. *Internet of Things*

The IoT ecosystem comprises Internet-connected physical gadgets, cars, household appliances and other objects. The IoT can be incorporated in smart grids and other sectors. The existing centralized Internet infrastructure makes it impossible to meet IoT development objectives, such as the confidentiality of sensitive information and the trustworthiness of interactions between multiple devices. As a result, the integration of the IoT with Blockchain has become an unavoidable trend, and smart contracts will aid in automating complicated workflows, encouraging resource sharing, saving money and ensuring safety and efficiency (Ayed 2017).

2.2.2.4. *Energy*

Blockchain could power a decentralized energy system and implement smart contracts for power generation and trade in order to develop decentralized energy trading markets, and improve energy and consumption efficiency. Exergy (Exergy n.d.) is a Blockchain consortium platform that offers suitable energy markets for power trades via the existing power grid. Sun Exchange (Sun Exchange n.d.) is a marketplace based on Blockchain that allows customers to buy solar cells and then rent them out to organizations and communities in the sunniest regions in the world (mainly Africa). The income of its members is based on electricity generated through its solar cells. Sun Exchange will be responsible for the collection and distribution of monthly rent. Knirsch et al. (2018) provided a selection of trustworthy, autonomous and anonymity charging points affordability and range to electric vehicles.

2.2.3. *Programming languages and platforms*

Smart contracts may be created and deployed on a variety of Blockchain platforms. Platforms differ in their features. In this section, two common platforms, Ethereum and Hyperledger Fabric, are discussed.

– Ethereum: on the Ethereum platform, applications execute precisely as designed, with no downtime, censorship or other issues such as fraud or intervention from a third party. The Ethereum Virtual Computer (EVM) is a Turing-complete VM, which is used to implement bytecode (as previously stated, Solidity compiles bytecode). Ethereum apps are powered by Ether, the platform's proprietary cryptographic token. Ether is used in the following ways: it is exchanged as an electronic asset similar to Bitcoin, and it is also used to reward nodes for completed calculations (ConsenSys 2016).

– Hyperledger Fabric: this is a distributed ledger technology. The Linux Foundation hosts Hyperledger Fabric. It offers high levels of discretion, robustness, customization and sustainability. It was created to allow for configurable solutions of specific parts, while also addressing the economic ecosystem's intricacy and complexities. Container technology is used by Hyperledger Fabric to store smart contracts called "chaincode".

Ethereum smart contract scripts, as previously indicated in section 2.1, are created in a bytecode language, which is based on stack and implemented in EVM. Ethereum smart contracts may be created in a number of high-level programming languages. Following that, the programs will be compiled into EVM bytecodes, which will be executed. Hyperledger Fabric generates SCs in a variety of languages, including Go and Java.

2.3. Quantitative analysis

Quantitative research is based on scientific inquiry and relies on data that has been observed or measured to answer questions about the sample population. The findings of quantitative research explain what is and is not relevant to, or impacts, a certain population. It also provides answers to inquiries about the frequency of a phenomenon or the extent to which it affects the sample, and also provides useful data for product design, such as information on user demands, behavior patterns and use cases.

We examined the Scopus database for research published until November 1, 2021. Studies on Blockchain smart contracts have been published not only in medical publications, but also in journals from other fields such as IT, law, engineering, economics and business administration. As a result, given its comprehensive coverage of journals in both the scientific and social sciences, we chose the Scopus database as the source of papers for this study.

We employed four processes to conduct a comprehensive quantitative review: discovering possible research, screening out irrelevant studies, confirming relevant studies and assessing chosen papers.

In the first phase of selecting suitable research, we conducted a preliminary search for papers that had a term like "Blockchain smart contract" in their titles, abstracts or keywords. This phase yielded a total of 5,873 prospective studies. In a separate search, we limited these studies to those that had key phrases like "Blockchain smart contract healthcare" in their titles, abstracts or keywords. This resulted in a total of 373 prospective studies.

In the second phase, a filter was applied to remove the articles in press, which yielded the 356 documents out of 373 documents. The Scopus database also shows articles in press, which means that the articles are not yet published online but are in the production stage.

We investigated the types of document, titles, abstracts and keywords in the third phase of validation, and filtered out 354 studies that fulfilled the criterion of our search for documents published in the English language alone.

We studied the distribution of the 354 articles by publication year, language, place of origin, journal and yearly average number of citations in the fourth phase of evaluation. The articles' nations of origin were investigated by determining the nationalities of the organizations to which the authors belonged. If an article had two writers working for organizations in two distinct nations, the country of origin was determined to be two countries. The top 10 articles were determined using the yearly average number of citations of the 464 articles. By adjusting for the effects of time after publication, the yearly average number of citations can more effectively represent the degree of influence of each piece on other research than the overall number of citations. For example, an article published in 2016 is more likely to have been referenced than one published in 2019. As a result, we used the yearly average number of citations to rank the 354 papers.

2.3.1. *Results*

First, the number of articles has dramatically increased since 2016. These articles began being published in 2016. In 2016, only one article was published. From 2017, the number of articles continuously increased in the domain of Blockchain-based smart contracts for healthcare. Figure 2.3 shows the rise in the number of articles from 2016 to 2021.

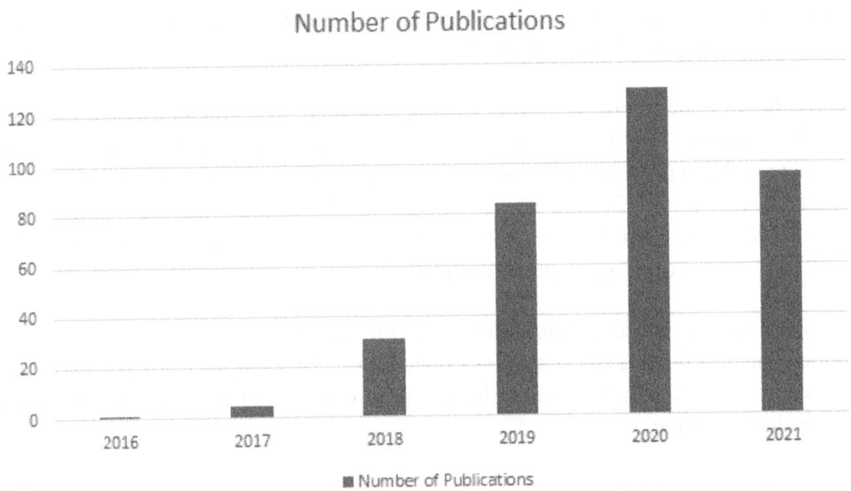

Figure 2.3. *Number of publications*

India, the United States, China, the United Kingdom and Australia are the top 5 countries in terms of the number of articles published. India has the maximum number of articles, i.e. 82, which constitutes around 23.1% of the selected articles for review. Figure 2.4 shows the top 5 countries.

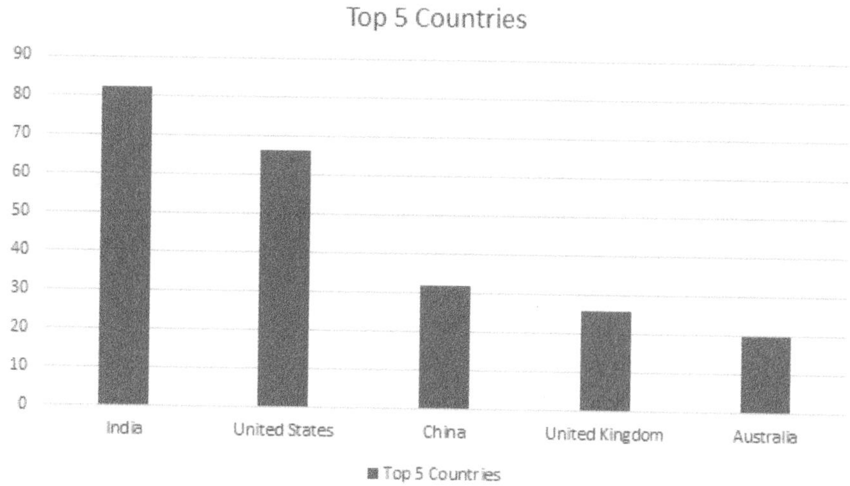

Figure 2.4. *Top 5 countries in terms of publications*

IEEE Access, PervasiveHealth: Pervasive Computing Technologies for Healthcare, Lecture Notes in Computer Science including subseries Lecture Notes in Artificial Intelligence and Lecture Notes in Bioinformatics, Lecture Notes in Networks and Systems, Advances in Intelligent Systems and Computing are the top 5 five sources in terms of number of publications. IEEE Access has the maximum number of documents, i.e. 22. Figure 2.5 shows the top 5 sources.

The goal of quantitative research is to develop information and understanding of the social world. Social scientists, especially communication scholars, employ quantitative research to examine events or occurrences that effect humans. The above quantitative analysis allows researchers to execute basic or complicated studies, such as displaying data linkages, calculating averages or percentages or using inferential statistics to draw broad generalizations about a huge population. This article will be useful to academicians and practitioners who are interested in Blockchain technology for building smart contracts and seeking collaboration opportunities with other academicians and research institutions by carefully collecting, categorizing and assessing research publications related to Blockchain-based smart contracts.

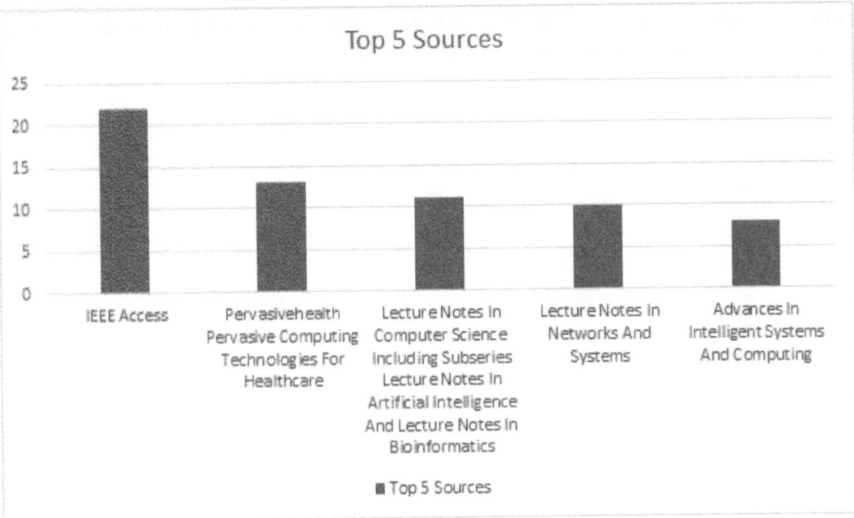

Figure 2.5. *Top 5 sources in terms of number of publications*

2.4. Role of smart contracts in healthcare

2.4.1. *Health Insurance*

Smart contracts possess the ability to remove various inconsistencies in the current setup and may be used on a regular basis in medical insurance. Whenever users use smart contracts to acquire coverage, all policy details are recorded in the user identity quickly. This content is again recorded on the Blockchain.

They may reduce the burden involved with completing paperwork in claim processes. If an insuree has to undertake a clinical procedure covered by the medical policy, the SC will be activated instantly. Therefore, the money through the insurance organization's wallet will be transferred to the medical facility. This mechanism avoids any inefficiencies and inconvenience, while still enabling the correct reimbursement for health services. As a result, all activities between participants will be accelerated, and the operation would be completed on time.

2.4.2. *Healthcare*

SCs allow data and documents to be recorded on a Blockchain system. This means that if a person has to move through one clinic to the next, they can do it quickly, without needing to complete multiple forms. On the Blockchain network, records may then be seen by the patient's selected physician.

A number of records containing health information are used by health facilities and medical agencies. These, nevertheless, may be too limited to enable the worldwide distribution of possibly existing information. This data can take a while to get the rightful owner and could be hacked if smart contracts and Blockchain are not used.

If patient details are saved in an SC and maintained on the Blockchain, these records can be accessed by the clinics and academic institutions all over the world. With sufficient acceptance, a user can enter into any clinic in the world for medication, and the organization would have quick accessibility to personal records provided they presented their secret key.

2.4.3. *Telemedicine*

Telehealth is a fast-growing healthcare profession. It allows clinicians and caregivers to connect with their clients using digital equipment such as cell phones as well as other IoT devices. Its major function is to provide treatment for the chronically sick. Practitioners can use videoconferencing to track treatment adherence and obtain actual information on their clients' health. These technology advancements help to improve patient results by enhancing connectivity and lowering operational costs.

Telemedicine has downsides due to the fact that the procedures entailed are a frequent target for cyber criminals. SCs protect the security and confidentiality of health records and other important patient documentation. To exchange and maintain data, SCs may be applied on a wide level and saved on the Blockchain. They could also help with record upkeep and make sure that critical medical details are kept secure and openly.

2.5. Example of smart contracts

2.5.1. *Simple open auction*

The basic principle behind the below Solidity simple auction contract is that everyone can submit offers throughout the auction time. Bids already involve the transfer of funds/ether to tie bidders to their bid. If the top offer is increased, the prior highest bidder receives a refund. After the bidding time has ended, the contract must be explicitly contacted in order for the recipient to collect their money –

contracts cannot trigger automatically. The below-mentioned example is written in Solidity.

```
pragma solidity >=0.4.22 <0.6.0;
contract AuctionSimple {
    address payable public beneficiary;

    uint public AuctionCompleteTime;

    address public LargestBidder;

    uint public LargestBid;

    mapping(address => uint) pendingReturns;

    bool ended;

    event LargestBidIncreased(uint amount, address bidder);

    event CompleteAuction(uint amount, address winner);

    constructor(

        uint _biddingTime,

        address payable _beneficiary

    ) public {

        beneficiary = _beneficiary;

        AuctionCompleteTime = now + _biddingTime;

    }

  function bid() public payable {

            now <= AuctionCompleteTime,

            "Auction already ended."

        );
```

```
        require(
            msg.value > LargestBid,
            "There already is a higher bid."
        );
    if (LargestBid != 0) {
            pendingReturns[LargestBidder]
LargestBid;
        }
        LargestBidder = msg.sender;
        LargestBid = msg.value;
        emit LargestBidIncreased(msg.sender, msg.value);
    }
    function withdraw() public returns (bool) {
        uint amount = pendingReturns[msg.sender];
        if (amount > 0) {
            pendingReturns[msg.sender] = 0;
            if (!msg.sender.send(amount)) {
                pendingReturns[msg.sender] = amount;
                return false;
            }
        }
        return true;
    }
```

```
    function auctionEnd() public {
        require(now >= AuctionCompleteTime);
        require(!ended);
        ended = true;
        emit CompleteAuction(LargestBidder, LargestBid);
        beneficiary.transfer(LargestBid);
    }
}
```

Smart Contract 2.1.

The function bid() places a bid on the auction using the value supplied. If the auction is not won, the value will be reimbursed. The method withdraw() removes an overbid bid, while the function auctionEnd() closes the auction and delivers the greatest bid to the recipient.

2.5.2. *Voting*

```
pragma solidity ^0.4.22;
contract Ballot {
    struct Balloter {
        bool castedcastvote;
        uint weight;
        address delegate;
        uint castvote;
    }
```

```
    struct Selection {
        bytes32 name;
        uint countCastvote;
    }
    address public chief;
    mapping(address => Balloter) public balloter;
    Selection[] public Selections;
    constructor(bytes32[] NameSelection) public {
        chief = msg.messenger;
        balloter[chief].weight = 1;
        for (uint i = 0; i < NameSelection.length; i++) {
            Selections.push(Selection({
                name: NameSelection[i],
                countCastvote: 0
            }
)
);
      }
   }
   function Balloterights(address balloter) public {
      require(
         msg.messenger == chief,
         "only chief has access to give the castvote."
```

```
    );
    require(
        !balloter[balloter].castedcastvote,
        "already castedcastvote."
    );
    require(balloters[balloter].weight == 0);
    balloter[balloter].weight = 1;
}
function delegate(address to) public {
    // assigns reference
    Balloter storage messenger = balloter[msg.messenger];
    require(!messenger.castedcastvote, "finish voting.");
    require(to != msg.messenger, "Self-delegation is not permitted.");
        to = balloter[to].delegate;
        require(to != msg.messenger, "Delegation loop discovered.");
    }
    messenger.castedcastvote = true;
    messenger.delegate = to;
    Balloter storage delegate_ = balloter[to];
    if (delegate_.castedcastvote) {

        Selections[delegate_.castvote].countCastvote += messenger.weight;
    } else {
```

```
            delegate_.weight += messenger.weight;
        }
    }
    function castvote(uint Selection) public {
        Balloter storage messenger = balloter[msg.messenger];
        require(!messenger.castedcastvote, "finish voting.");
        messenger.castedcastvote = true;
        messenger.castvote = Selection;
        Selections[Selection].countCastvote += messenger.weight;
    }
    function SelectionWin() public view
            returns (uint SelectionWin_)
    {
        uint winningCountCastvote = 0;
        for (uint p = 0; p < Selections.length; p++) {
            if (Selections[p].countCastvote > winningCountCastvote) {
                winningCountCastvote = Selections[p].countCastvote;
                SelectionWin_ = p;
            }
        }
    }
    function NameWinner() public view
```

```
        returns (bytes32 NameWinner_)
    {
      NameWinner_ = Selections[SelectionWin()].name;
    }
}
```

Smart Contract 2.2.

The function contract ballot declares a new complex type for variables. It symbolizes one balloter. A single Selection is a type of struct Selection. Mapping(address => Balloter) defines a state variable that holds a Balloter struct for each address. The function Balloterights(address balloter) does the following operations: If the initial argument of require responds to false, then operation is terminated and all modifications to the configuration and Ether amounts are reversed. This can be used to utilize all of the gas in prior EVM iterations, but it no longer does. To ensure that services are called correctly, it is usually a good strategy to use require. We may also give an explanation for what went wrong as a second argument. The function delegate() is used to assign a castvote to the balloter. The castvote() function returns the castvote (including castvotes cast) for Selection Selections[Selection].name. The function SelectionWin() calculates the winning Selection by considering the account of all previous castvotes. The NameWinner() function runs the SelectionWin() function to retrieve the winner's index from the Selections array and callback the winner's name.

2.5.3. *Patient record*

```
pragma solidity ^0.4.19;

contract RecordPatientData {

  // Part 1 Enums

  enum Gender { Male, Female }
```

```
// Part 2 Structs
struct Patient {
    uint age;
    bytes32 name;
    Gender gender;
}

// Part 3 State Variables
uint id;
Patient private patient;
address public ownerData;
// ** Part 4 ** Events **
event GetNamePatient(address sender);

// Part 5 Modifiers
modifier onlyOwner() {
    require(msg.sender == ownerData);
    _;
}
// Part 6 Functions
function RecordPatientData() public {
    dataOwner= msg.sender;
}
```

```
function getDataPatient() public returns (bytes32) {
    GetNamePatient(msg.sender);
    return patient.name;
}
    function setPatientName(bytes32 name) public onlyOwner {
    patient.name = name;
}

}
```

Smart Contract 2.3.

Part 1 discusses an enum that is used to declare the patient's gender and Part 2 describes a struct. Part 3 discusses the state variables. A state variable merely indicates the status of a certain record for a patient. In the above program, there are three state variables: a unique id, the patient for the data and the state variable for the smart contract address that owns this patient history. Function RecordPatientData() gives the address of the generating smart contract to dataOwner, a state variable that can be used later. Part 4 describes events and Part 5 describes modifiers. Part 6 discusses functions, which are nothing more than constructors, getters and setters.

2.6. Challenges related to smart contracts

Smart contracts, being an emerging technology in its early stages, are now afflicted by a plethora of difficulties and roadblocks. This section will describe the issues with smart contracts, as well as current research developments.

2.6.1. *Contract vulnerabilities*

– Transaction-ordering dependence (TOD): each block includes numerous activities, and the miner determines the order that they are completed in. TOD occurs when a large number of reliant actions execute the same contract in a manner in which the miners have influence over the sequence wherein the transactions are performed.

– Timestamp dependence: the miners calculate the date and time for the transaction generated. They may change the timestamp by a few seconds if other miners approve the transaction they provided. The problem comes from the fact that certain smart contracts use a time as a triggering event, such as a payment system, and thus an adversary might be altered.

– Mishandled exceptions: once a contract communicates with another, the present operation pauses for the call to complete before proceeding. The caller may or may not be notified of this exception. To verify that the call was completed, the responder should expressly check the callee's callback function. Nevertheless, if the client refuses to properly examine the callback function, it may lead to potential dangers.

– Re-entrancy vulnerability: once a contract communicates with another, the present operation pauses for the call to complete before proceeding. Also, because the fallback method enables an intruder to re-enter the caller's method, an intruder may take advantage of the sender's initial point to conduct repeated calls, culminating in loops of invocations that get many reimbursements and drain the balance. One of the most well-known re-entry vulnerabilities is the Decentralized Autonomous Organizations (DAO) attack (CoinDesk n.d.).

Some security analysis tools are being developed to address contract issues. Since many contract problems are caused by a lexical mismatch among developers' knowledge of the underlying executing meanings smart contracts, Luu et al. (2016) developed Oyente, a symbolic processing tool, to identify possible security bugs in Ethereum smart contracts. Oyente identified 8,833 Ethereum smart contracts as susceptible out of 19366, including the DAO bug. Its analysis is divided into two steps: first, it symbolically examines the dependency structure of the contract in order to elicit precise linguistic metadata from the program. After this, it analyses violation and different activities to see if they capture enough criteria to determine if a property is valid or not. Many flaws, like transaction reordering, repetitive calls, unsafe code patterns and so on, can be analyzed by Securify. Manticore (GitHub n.d.) seems to be another regular expression technique for evaluating binary and smart contracts. It is capable of capturing a program execution trail for each produced input.

2.6.2. *Privacy and legal issues*

There are two types of smart contract privacy concerns: 1) contract data privacy; 2) reliable data feeds privacy. Not only events, but also contract-related metadata (especially for content on the public Blockchain), including such bytecode, activation arguments and so on, are now publicly accessible. As a result, it is a significant task to keep essential functions/methods hidden, use cryptography and prevent data that should not have been made public from being revealed. The contracts layer is primarily responsible for smart contract legal concerns.

In addition to the issues described above, there are numerous other issues based on the architecture and contract layers. Poor smart contract design mechanisms result in an increase in contract running expenses and minimizes running efficiency on the operations layer. Malevolent intelligent agents on the intelligence layer may profit from their malicious conduct and so on.

2.6.3. *Immutability issue*

The immutability property is a key aspect of smart contracts. Indeed, once a smart contract is launched, no one can modify the code. However, the disadvantage of the immutability notion in smart contracts is that in the event of any flaws in the code, the immutability characteristic of a smart contract prohibits them from being corrected. Similarly, if circumstances change (e.g. the parties have mutually decided to modify the conditions of their commercial transaction, or if the legislation changes, etc.), there is no simple solution to modify a smart contract. To overcome the immutability issue, lengthy and perhaps expensive evaluations of the smart contract by experts prior to its implementation in a Blockchain are necessary.

2.7. Conclusion

Due to the tremendous advancement of Blockchain technology, creating SCs has been a prominent subject for both research and businesses. The immutability and irreversibility of smart contracts can encourage users to exchange currency, stocks and proprietary information, as well as other commodities in a clear, conflict-free way, without the participation of a foreign entity. This chapter provides an introduction to Blockchain technology, along with some characteristics and applications. It also provides in depth details about Blockchain smart contracts, its operating mechanism and applications in different domains. It provides details about the different platforms for smart contract and concludes with the research challenges in implementing smart contracts.

2.8. References

Ayed, A. (2017). A conceptual secure blockchain-based electronic voting system. *International Journal of Network Security & Its Applications (IJNSA)*, 9. DOI: 10.5121/ijnsa.2017.9301.

Bitcoin (n.d.). Bitcoin: A peer-to-peer electronic cash system [Online]. Available at: https://bitcoin.org/en/bitcoin-paper [Accessed 12 July 2022].

CoinDesk (n.d.). What is a DAO? [Online]. Available at: https://www.coindesk.com/learn/what-is-a-dao/ [Accessed 12 July 2022].

CoinDesk (2016a). State of Blockchain Q1 2016: Blockchain funding overtakes Bitcoin [Online]. Available at: https://www.coindesk.com/markets/2016/05/11/state-of-blockchain-q1-2016-blockchain-funding-overtakes-bitcoin/ [Accessed 12 July 2022].

CoinDesk (2016b). Making sense of Blockchain smart contracts [Online]. Available at: https://www.coindesk.com/markets/2016/06/04/making-sense-of-blockchain-smart-contracts/ [Accessed 12 July 2022].

ConsenSys (2016). Ethereum, gas, fuel, & fees [Online]. Available at: https://media.consensys.net/ethereum-gas-fuel-and-fees-3333e17fe1dc [Accessed 12 July 2022].

ConsenSys Mesh (n.d.). Ethereum investments, research, & protocols [Online]. Available at: https://mesh.xyz/ [Accessed 12 July 2022].

Exergy (n.d.). Exergy [Online]. Available at: https://exergy.energy/ [Accessed 12 July 2022].

Gatteschi, V., Lamberti, F., Demartini, C., Pranteda, C., Santamaría, V. (2018). Blockchain and smart contracts for insurance: Is the technology mature enough? *Future Internet*, 10(2), 20. DOI: 10.3390/FI10020020.

GitHub (n.d.). Manticore: Symbolic execution tool [Online]. Available at: https://github.com/trailofbits/manticore [Accessed 12 July 2022].

Idelberger, F., Governatori, G., Riveret, R., Sartor, G. (2016). Evaluation of logic-based smart contracts for blockchain systems. *Lecture Notes in Computer Science (Including Subseries Lecture Notes in Artificial Intelligence and Lecture Notes in Bioinformatics)*, 9718, 167–183. DOI: 10.1007/978-3-319-42019-6_11/COVER.

Katal, A., Sethi, V., Lamba, S. (2021). Blockchain consensus algorithms: Study and challenges. *EAI/Springer Innovations in Communication and Computing*, 45–64. DOI: 10.1007/978-3-030-65691-1_4/COVER/.

Knirsch, F., Unterweger, A., Engel, D. (2018). Privacy-preserving Blockchain-based electric vehicle charging with dynamic tariff decisions. *Computer Science – Research and Development*, 33, 71–79. DOI: 10.1007/S00450-017-0348-5/TABLES/2.

Luu, L., Chu, D.H., Olickel, H., Saxena, P., Hobor, A. (2016). Making smart contracts smarter. *Proceedings of the ACM Conference on Computer and Communications Security*, 24–28 October, 254–269. DOI: 10.1145/2976749.2978309.

Maicher, L., de la Rosa, J.L., Gibovic, D. (2016). On intellectual property in online open innovation for SME by means of Blockchain and smart contracts. *World Open Innovation Conference* (*WOIC 2016*), Barcelona.

McCorry, P., Shahandashti, S.F., Hao, F. (2017). A smart contract for boardroom voting with maximum voter privacy. *Lecture Notes in Computer Science (Including Subseries Lecture Notes in Artificial Intelligence and Lecture Notes in Bioinformatics)*, 10322 LNCS, 357–375. DOI: 10.1007/978-3-319-70972-7_20.

Ojetunde, B., Shibata, N., Gao, J. (2019). Secure payment system utilizing MANET for disaster areas. *IEEE Transactions on Systems, Man, and Cybernetics: Systems*, 49, 2651–2663. DOI: 10.1109/TSMC.2017.2752203.

Pilkington, M. (2016). Blockchain technology: Principles and applications. *Research Handbooks on Digital Transformations*, 225–253. DOI: 10.4337/9781784717766.00019.

Sun Exchange (n.d.). Sun Exchange [Online]. Available at: https://thesunexchange.com/ [Accessed 12 July 2022].

Wang, S., Ouyang, L., Yuan, Y., Ni, X., Han, X., Wang, F.Y. (2019). Blockchain-enabled smart contracts: Architecture, applications, and future trends. *IEEE Transactions on Systems, Man, and Cybernetics: Systems*, 49, 2266–2277. DOI: 10.1109/TSMC.2019.2895123.

3

Blockchain-based Platforms for the Healthcare Industry

Blockchain technology is an emerging and promising technology, and studies conducted on Blockchain technology have shown a spurt. Some characteristic features of Blockchain, including transparency in data handling, better security insurance, open-sourcing, tracing and decentralization, make it a suitable innovation for undertaking the data imbalance issue in close to personal benefits announcing exchanges. A few efforts have been made at incorporating Blockchain technology in numerous business applications. Blockchain technology promises a decentralized trust giving an alternative to centralized data management and storage in the computerized or the digital environment. With the better and advanced models storage, tracking and management of payment systems and others, a significant change can be brought in the various industries and services. However, other than the decentralized storage property, Blockchain technology offers much more valuable propositions such as much more advanced and innovative investment models and crypto-economic currencies, radically new types of advanced models for governance which can generate further development in the age where digital platforms and business interactions have multi-stakeholders. Blockchain technology is a decentralized distributed digital ledger and is capable of transforming the underlying operating system that will administer the way our cities will function in the future. Blockchain is presently bringing a revolution in numerous industries like finance, healthcare, supply chain, insurance, registry and the Internet of Things (IoT). Numerous industries integrate Blockchain with their frameworks to benefit from the advantages of the Blockchain.

3.1. Introduction

The healthcare sector has its requirements for security and privacy to protect the patient's personal and medical information. We are living in a world where records and data are being stored on the cloud platforms and also the use of mobile health services has become common due to its easier access, therefore making the risk of

---

Chapter written by Dakshita NEGI, Anushree SHAH, Saurabh RAWAT and Tanupriya CHOUDHURY.

patient's information being compromised or leaked when shared through the Internet. Hence the requirements that the medical sector needs are in the form of "authentication, interoperability, data transfer of medical records and considerations for mobile healthcare system". In terms of revenue and employment, the healthcare sector has become one of the largest sectors according to the Indian Brand Equity Foundation (IBEF). The healthcare industry has been increasing at a vast pace and is not only limited to hospitals but also includes medical equipment, tourism, health insurance, clinics and now much more. Thus, there is notable growth in the market with the expansion of the healthcare sector.

US$ 327 billion will be the mark crossed by the healthcare industry by 2022. Growing at a compound annual growth rate (CAGR) of 16–17%, the hospital industry will see three folds in the US$ 133.44 billion by 2023. The changed lifestyle of the people and increment in the mean income of people and government and insurance policies has resulted in increased health awareness among the people, leading to this massive increase in the healthcare industry (Gul et al. 2020).

3.2. Literature review

In the paper by Tripathi et al. (2019), the problem related to the medical sector has been discussed, which mainly includes security concerns and how Blockchain technology can significantly help in dealing with such issues. With the flood of medical records using EMR (Electronic Medical Records) and ICT, Blockchain is being used in many medical organizations. The paper discusses Blockchain technology and also the SHS-Smart Healthcare System and the challenges faced by it, further proposing a Blockchain-based SHS framework for analyzing and finding a solution to security and integrity issues.

The paper by A. Islam and Shin (2020) proposes a scheme in which an unmanned vehicle (UAV) collects healthcare data and stores it in the nearest server. Firstly, a relation is established by the UAV with the body sensor hives (BSHs) through a token and afterwards a shared key is generated with BSHs that further establishes a low-power secure communication. Once all the data is collected by UAV, it decrypts all of the encrypted data (shared key encryption is done) and works out a two-phase implementation. And thus, after validation, the UAV sends the data to the server which stores it in the Blockchain network. An even analysis is presented in the paper to show the practicability and the feasibility of the proposed scheme.

A smart healthcare business model observes the customers at the heart of the business, with the evolution of Blockchain technology. The paper by Gul et al. (2020) established that the suggested model can analyze the customer's level and then provide prizes, as per the regulations that have been set up by the participating organization. From the Internet of Medical Things, the model fetches data and then applies any related script in which the rewarding system exits. The model focuses on the customer and the business while relating technology to manage all of the stakeholders involved.

The paper by Ferrer-Gomila et al. (2019) provides an operational hybrid platform using a consensus mechanism that breaks the problem of partaking the sensitive information of the digital forensic medical evidence. The mechanism records the transparent history of the case and prevents the modification of the data by unauthorized users. Firstly, the digital evidence is encrypted before storing them in an online file storage system that is present in the Blockchain network. A dynamic agreement tool is applied to entertain the data in the Blockchain. Cryptography ensures secured access to digital data stored on various Blockchain nodes.

The complex nature of the modern healthcare system has made them costlier. The cost of the healthcare system can be reduced by befitting the application of insurance companies, amending record management and by using Blockchain technology as discussed in Tanwar et al. (2020). Breakthroughs in Blockchain technology have guided and helped to evolve transactions involving insurance billings, smart contracts and medical records. Using Blockchain in healthcare has many advantages, one of them being the capability to reform the interoperability of the data (healthcare and prescription), device tracking, etc. To prescribe the medication, it is important to know the patient's medical history, and Blockchain has helped to improve the medical sector framework in this case. Here, many solutions are explored to expand the boundaries of the healthcare system using Blockchain. To liquidate the Hyper-Ledger-based EHR sharing in the system that employs chain code, for correcting data accessibility among healthcare providers, helping in the stimulation of the environment, the Access Control Policy Algorithm is examined. The proposed scheme uses Blockchain technology to improve efficiency and security instead of the traditional system that uses a client-server architecture.

The paper by Abd-alrazaq et al. (2020) discusses the Covid-19 situation currently in the world and how we can use Blockchain technology to mitigate the challenges that are being faced due to the virus. The paper shows various properties of the Blockchain that are generally used in the healthcare sector and the applications that can be used to help government authorities to face the challenges due to the virus. In the fight against the Covid-19 virus, Blockchain technologies are expected to play a significant role.

The paper by Huang et al. (2020) offers a privacy-preserving scheme based on Blockchain technology to ensure safe sharing of the data between the patient and the medical research institution. This scheme not only accomplishes data availability but also consistency between the patient and the institution. A zero-knowledge proof is provided to make sure that the patients' medical information meets up to the requirements of the research institution, and further a proxy re-encryption technology is used by the institution to decrypt the intermediate cypher text. This scheme can also implement a distributed consensus based on the PBFT algorithm for the transaction purpose between the patient and the institution.

When talking about the traditional medical management systems, certain drawbacks can be addressed by the advancement in cloud-assisted electronic health systems. But at the same time, ensuring the integrity of the electronic health records (EHR) along with guaranteeing the privacy and traceability of the EHR while sharing is not easy. Thus, the paper by Huang et al. (2020) proposes a Blockchain-based eHealth system BCES to check the manipulation of the healthcare records. Every handling of the data consumers together with every outsourcing control of the hospitals, in the intended system, will be penned in a pattern of a transaction in the Blockchain in the form of storage that will ensure traceability. Also, the proxy re-encrypted system that is used to gain access control of the medical data and the auditors will recognize any sort of behavior or activity that can threaten the integrity of EHRs. This scheme, due to its security analysis and performance evaluation, has stood out to be secure and efficient.

The paper by Negi et al. (2021) presents a healthcare data managing system that focuses on the patient (patient-centric) using the Blockchain technology as storage to help with maintaining privacy. In today's world, cyber-attacks have become a common thing especially in the cloud. The data stored on the cloud has always been an attraction to them, and the healthcare data has not been an exception to this. Attacks on healthcare data can be very damaging to organizations in the medical sector. Decentralization which is enabled by the peer-to-peer network makes the storing and running of the healthcare as well as the data in the cloud possible. The Blockchain, because of its decentralized character, guarantees accountability and integrity. Cryptographic functions encrypt patients' data and ensure pseudo-anonymity. The cost efficiency of the smart contracts and data processing strategies are employed.

A Blockchain-based architecture is a potential solution to a lot of problems related to the contemporary e-Healthcare networks, discussed by Choudhury et al. (2021). In the modern e-healthcare systems, human recognition activity (HRA) can be said to be one of the most challenging tasks when it comes to monitoring patients who are affected by either disabilities or mental illness and require assistance, and protecting several distinct devices that are connected to the Internet – Internet of Things – is a major issue. Also, numerous activities that are performed by the human being at a time in the diverse healthcare environment decrease the quality of those activities.

We are well aware that the EHRs have been playing an important role in the e-healthcare system where the exchange of a patient's medical records by means of a portal is assigned by medical professionals, but there are security issues due to the lack of integrity and confidentiality. The paper by Benil and Jasper (2020) has proposed the Elliptical Curve Certificate less Aggregate Cryptography Signature scheme (EC-ACS), for securing the EHRs by verifying and reviewing the information in the Medical Server Cloud (MSC) by use of the Blockchain technology. For sharing and storing the data in the medical cloud storage, Elliptical Curve Cryptography (ECC) is used for encrypting the medical data and Certificate less Aggregate Signature (CAS) for generating a digital signature. Security and privacy are promised by this scheme, and it also safeguards confidential information from malicious activities in the cloud health storage.

The privacy of sensitive medical data can be compromised when they are shared beyond the scope of the institutions. A Blockchain-based solution has been proposed in Hussein et al. (2018) to resolve the challenges that are related to access control and handling the data. To improve security, the system is equipped with discrete wavelet transform and to upgrade the queuing optimization technique, a genetic algorithm is deployed. Verifying the user becomes fast with the use of this cryptographic key generator as it improves the immunity and the access control of the system. This design allows accountability as the number of users are known and the Blockchain keeps a record of the user's actions. The sharing of the data is allowed only when cryptographic keys and identities are known.

In the paper by Nguyen et al. (2020), an analysis of the patient's data that has been encrypted using Blockchain technology is presented. Nowadays, because of advancements occurring in technology, data sharing has become a challenge; on the one hand, the compatibility can be compromised by using heterogeneous data, while on the other hand, the distinctive use of the medical terminologies has limited data comprehension. We have seen that authorized users and centralized data storage have been targets for attackers, and the establishment of the health records over a data-sharing network can be troublesome. For data discovery and access, the concord mechanism is used to substantiate the proof of word and inter-operability. "The approach offered by the paper gives a centralized trust-based source for network consensus and compute consensus proof of semantic and structural interoperability".

In the paper by Dagher et al. (2018), a Blockchain-assumed framework has been alleged for an interoperable, secure and efficient siege to data by authorized users while preserving the patient's information. This framework was proposed since despite increasing the security of EHRs and the efforts made by cities all over the globe to form a "smart city infrastructure", a person's personal information is at the risk of getting leaked. Earlier, the solutions which were provided caused the information to be out of the reach of the patients. The data management systems that are present struggle to balance between data confidentiality and the necessity for the patient and provider to interact with the data regularly. Advanced cryptographic techniques for likewise security, Ancile uses smart contracts in an Ethereum-based Blockchain, for access control and data complication. The paper examines how Ancile would cater to the diverse needs of the patients, professionals and third parties and how this framework could address the longstanding privacy and security problems.

The paper by Chen et al. (2019) talks about a Blockchain-based encryption scheme for EHRs. Leakage of data in EHRs can result in the patient's information being jeopardized and since most of these records once uploaded do not change, the Blockchain technology can potentially be used to enable data sharing. In the Blockchain network, we have the index of the EHR stored in the form of complex logical expressions for the user to use these expressions and find the index later. Also, the user has complete control over to whom their EHRs are visible because only the index is migrated to the Blockchain to enable propagation. The performance scheme is estimated in two aspects, one for pulling the document IDs from the EHRs and the second for yielding the transactions in the smart contracts in the Ethereum.

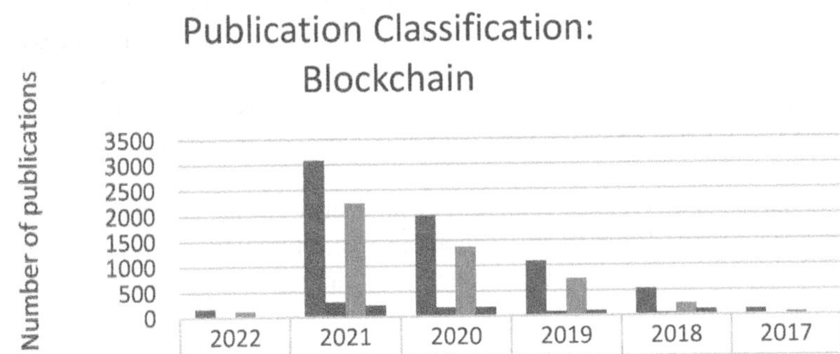

	2022	2021	2020	2019	2018	2017
Total Publications	157	3072	1986	1079	526	122
Review articles	13	300	174	79	44	10
Research articles	120	2237	1370	734	236	61
Book chapters	12	232	181	94	117	10

Figure 3.1. *Publication classification for Blockchain. For a color version this figure, see www.iste.co.uk/choudhury/blockchain.zip*

GuardHealth discussed in the paper Comput et al. (2020) refers to a secure, decentralized and efficient Blockchain system used for sharing and privacy of data. When managing sensitive health records, GuardHealth seeks to achieve a share of data, preserving of data, authentication and confidentiality. Here the sharing of data without permission cannot be done as the system makes use of smart contracts and Blockchain to secure data sharing and storing. A model is used for accurately keeping the trust of the users, with the implementation of state-of-the-art graph neural network (GNN) for illegal actions. For smart healthcare systems, the proposed scheme in security analysis and experiments has proved to be ideal. Figure 3.1 shows the publication classification of Blockchain technology. The graph shows that the technology is gaining publicity, and in the coming years, Blockchain would be seen in many verticals of the IT industry.

3.3. Blockchain technology

Blockchain is described as a distributed and digital ledger system that gives the concept of transparency and user privacy. The concept of Blockchain was introduced for the financial and business industry at first but now due to its features, it is being applied to other sectors as well where security has now become an issue (Rawat and Sah 2012). Blockchain technology is dependent on the value-to-value architecture where the data (in form of blocks) is joined using cryptography technique (chain). Figure 3.2 shows the publication classification of Blockchain in healthcare from 2017 to 2022. The graph below shows that Blockchain technology soon will be adopted on a large scale in the healthcare industry.

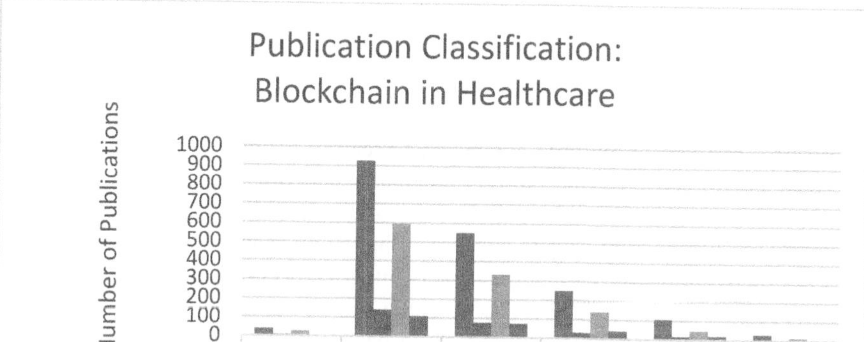

	2022	2021	2020	2019	2018	2017
Total Publications	37	925	548	250	104	29
Review articles	7	141	76	29	16	3
Research articles	26	596	331	140	47	14
Book chapters	2	108	72	40	19	3

Figure 3.2. *Publication classification for Blockchain in the healthcare industry. For a color version this figure, see www.iste.co.uk/choudhury/blockchain.zip*

3.3.1. *Uses of Blockchain in the healthcare sector*

Blockchain technology has been extensively studied and researched thus, the features of the Blockchain can be used to provide a solution in the healthcare industry for the related matter.

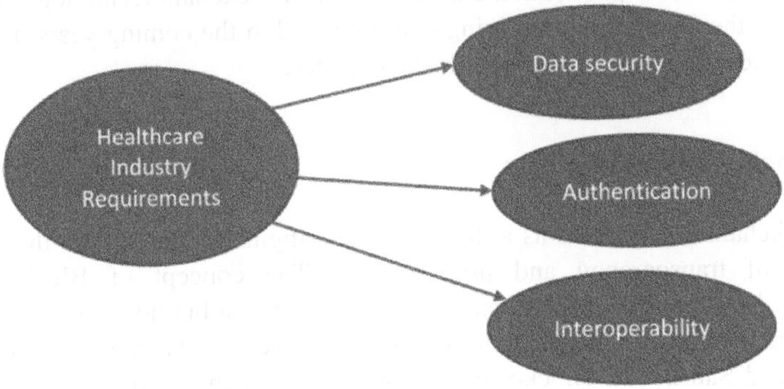

Figure 3.3. *Healthcare industry*

3.3.1.1. *Security*

We need to have a proper technology or network to protect and secure the records, and at present, the methods which are being used are not effective. "Data security, integrity and immutability" are the main features of Blockchain technology. Blockchain by the use of a secure decentralized ledger can offer security as it stores the data in multiple computers instead of a single computer. By having the data distributed over the entire Blockchain network, we have the same data stored in many computers. Now we cannot have any third party or malicious actor changing the information or data as the data has to be changed in all the computers over the network. Also, data security and integrity becomes the primary concern when applied to smart devices and cloud infrastructure. By providing "data provenance, auditing and control for cloud-based server", Blockchain technology can allow safe data sharing among the devices and over the Internet that deposits the medical data, which is shared by using the smart contracts and access protocol implementations.

3.3.1.2. *Interoperability*

Interoperability can be defined as the operation of transferring and sharing data between varied sources. Because of the use of centralized data storage in the medical sector, it was not possible to use the feature of interoperability that is required in the healthcare industry. "Centralized data storage" can be problematic to the providers because it means storing the data in a single central database thus hampering the quality and quantity of the medical data and researches, having slow access to the patient data, and also the disintegration of the healthcare data (Sah et al. 2018).

The decentralized storage feature of the Blockchain can be very useful for better security and authentication of the data stored in the systems (Khanna et al. 2020a). Decentralized storage is the process in which there is a breakdown of the records in the storage from the single server to numerous servers by the means of a Blockchain ledger. In this way, we can have an enhanced quality and quantity of the data and also faster access to the patient's information.

3.3.1.3. *Authentication*

Blockchain by the means of its decentralized feature makes sure the authentication of the patient record that is present in the blocks of the Blockchain. The authentication process is achieved by a private key which in turn is connected to a public key to initialize the operation of creation, modification and checking of the information in the Blockchain. In the software, a Bitcoin wallet is associated with the Bitcoin address and stores these keys. By the use of the cryptographic scheme, the software applications which are usually used for bitcoin and cryptocurrency can be determined for authentication purposes.

3.4. Blockchain applications that can be useful for treating the medical sector problems

3.4.1. *Smart contracts*

Employing smart contracts, the user can form or create agreements between the buyer and the seller, by using Blockchain technology. Smart contracts, stored in Blockchain network, encrypt and convert the transaction into legal documents for legal services. These smart contracts consist of the scripts that are present in the Blockchain network, and they can be traced or identified by their unique address. By means of these smart contracts, we can establish a fair exchange among the parties while having minimum communication between them, in a decentralized manner. Thus, by this, the user can form their document without the need of a legal representative thus removing the challenges including both financial and time-wise, and making a better transfer of the resources or transaction.

3.4.2. *Fraud detection*

It is the process that verifies the document or the data in the system to check if there is any kind of tempering with information or malicious conduct, for example, the false comments and ratings which are given in the online review system in the form of bad-mouthing as well as the scams happening in the financial industry in the form of loan applications, etc. The idea of fraud detection can also be applied in the concept of crowdfunding where we have a bunch of people who are investing or buying stocks from the company. Blockchain technology can be used as a low-cost platform for registering shares and stocks and thus makes transactions quite secure, effective, efficient and easier.

3.4.3. *Identity verification*

The government system uses passports and the fingerprints of an individual to identify the person but Blockchain technology can provide an alternative to these identification methods (Khanna et al. 2020). Blockchains can identify the user, for example, using Blockchain in notarizing marriages, birth certificates and business contracts. For a person can prove their existence at a point in time, Blockchain would use its "distributed ledger" property and is further verified by a group of people by distributed nature of the Blockchain technology. For example, we can use Blockchain technology to validate marriages, birth contracts and business contracts.

3.5. Examples of healthcare platforms using Blockchain

3.5.1. *Data sharing using Gem Health Network*

As discussed earlier, the healthcare sector contains the records of patients and stores them in a centralized database, which can lead to issues such as data security and interoperability. If a patient needs the records when going through a specialized treatment either in another hospital, interstate or overseas, then the sharing of data becomes a problem. Every time a person sees another doctor, there is a need to form a new set of records and update several existing records, changing the communication protocols between the doctors, and also there is IT interference which is very time-consuming. Hence, there has been a solution given out for the problem by the Gem as Health Network that uses Ethereum Blockchain Technology and creates a shared network infrastructure. This network helps different professionals in the healthcare sector to access the same information and records of the patients, unlike the centralized database. Access to the latest treatment information (which is transparent and relevant) is only given to the authorized users. This helps in reducing the risk of neglecting a person's health issues due to misinformation or outdated health records.

For example, we have "Estonia who has collaborated with Guardtime that uses Blockchain technology. Thus, all the medical professionals, insurance companies and citizens can have access to the health records and treatments that have been performed in Estonia with the help of this technology, indicating a way in which Blockchain can be applied similarly as stated above".

3.5.2. *MeDshare*

MeDshare is a platform that is designed for sharing the data and records amongst medical professionals who store their data and records in a not so trustworthy environment. This system looks after the basic requirements in the medical sector such as maintaining the patient's privacy and risk of malicious activities on the medical records. MeDshare system uses the Blockchain technology providing data management, auditing and data provenance in the cloud-based environment among the companies. The system is designed in such a way that smart contracts and access control mechanisms are used to keep a track of data and to retract any malicious entity on the discovery of any kind of misbehavior in the system. The main aim of MeDshare is to provide the cloud providers (that store the medical records) with the capability of data management, auditing and data sharing to the medical industry without leaking the private information of the patient. This system is divided into four layers.

The first layer consists of the arrangements that are made for the users who are allowed to access the medical records.

The second layer (data query layer) consists of certain queries for accessing, processing, forwarding and responding to the requests. Here, the processes are broken down into two components – the first component being the system consisting of queries that are in control for generating requests, and the second component being the trigger that deciphers the transactions to and from the smart contracts.

The third layer (data structuring and provenance layer) involves processing of requests for accessing the information or data from the existing database amid various existents such as smart contracts, processing, authenticators, smart contracts, consensus nodes and Blockchain systems.

The fourth layer (existing database infrastructure) comprises the database that is executed by individuals to complete their tasks.

3.5.3. *OmniPHR*

OmniPHR is a model to handle the health records and information of the patients, giving them a clear view of the records stored across multiple health providers. It helps in keeping data up to date when it is stored in another system or modified by another provider. OmniPHR addresses the difference between the EHR and PHR. EHRs are set up according to the government standards that help to have uniform records over the country; this makes the records accurate and up to date. The EHRs are updated on a regular basis by medical professionals without the involvement of patients, unlike PHR in which the patients keep a track of their records. Here, OmniPHR creates a framework that helps in addressing this problem where the patients can have a comprehensive look at their records alongside the medical community that can have the desired accuracy of the records. It makes use of Blockchain technology with the focus of unifying data that has been distributed over several organizations. PHR would be stored in an organized way hierarchically, encrypted and distributed in data blocks present on the network. The user can access the OmniPHR records from anywhere – home, work or hospital. Some of the cloud computing features that are used, scalability, elasticity, middleware, encryption protocols, open standards, etc., are included in the model. The data flow of the model is data provided to open standards, and then it is changed by middleware technologies and encrypted and authorized by privacy and security modules before storing it in the series of repositories.

3.6. Blockchain during the Covid-19 pandemic

In today's world, the one which we refer to as the "global village", there has been a massive rise in health diseases and health issues, due to the sedentary lifestyle of the people and many factors including ecological and environmental factors. Recently, the Covid-19 virus has been wreaking havoc all across the globe since December 2019 leading to more than 54 million people affected and over 1300,000 deaths. This pandemic has overburdened healthcare systems all over the world. Because of its significant features which include decentralization, immutability, transparency and auditability, Blockchain has turned out to be very useful in technology.

> European Parliament Research Service considers the Blockchain technology to be one of the top 10 vital technologies to mitigate Covid-19 challenges.

The applications of the Blockchain technology used to mitigate Covid-19 challenges have been discussed in the paper by Abd-alrazaq et al. (2020). The paper jots down 10 cases of the Blockchain technology to tackle the situations that have emerged due to the coronavirus, out of which six studies discuss contact tracing, i.e. the process that traces down those who were in close contact with the people who tested positive with Covid-19, and the remaining four studies discuss the application of immunity passports, which will show that a person is free from the disease because either they have already been infected with the disease or have been vaccinated with the Covid-19 vaccine.

The tracing of Covid-19-positive cases in the community was the primary requirement of the authorities to keep the outbreak of the virus in check. With knowing or having the records of people who were tested positive with Covid-19 and their close contacts, we could identify the "hotspot" areas and try to prevent the further spread of the virus. The technology that was being used was not giving assurance in preserving privacy with the centralized design of the technology giving the government the ability to do mass surveillance. Now Blockchain having a decentralized system is being used to provide better protection for government documents. Similarly, immunity passports, also known as immunity certificates or recovery certificates, given to the positive patients after they have fully recovered from the infection and Covid-19 diagnoses, make use of Blockchain technology in storing and sharing patient's information to only authorized users. For accessing sensitive documents, smart contracts are also being used in the form of an extra layer. The general properties of the Blockchain, which includes the applications for remote monitoring, tracking status and identity verification, are now being used.

3.7. Conclusion

The growing demand for health has led to the development of hospitals and medical institutions further leading to an increase in medical data and the need for managing it. Thus, we have discussed Blockchain technology in association with the medical sector. Health records including the personal details of the patients are to be kept confidential. These records are saved in "medical clouds" but can be misused by the other parties, for example by deleting the original data or modifying it. The problems related to the healthcare industry and how they can hamper technological advancements in the industry preventing it from growing have also been discussed in this chapter. Blockchain due to its various properties can be a solution to these problems, and Blockchain-based systems seem to exhibit higher robustness, scalability and immunity that allows secure data sharing and data privacy. Blockchain technology has now gained great attention in many countries and companies all over the world.

3.8. References

Abd-Alrazaq, A.A., Alajlani, M., Alhuwail, D., Erbad, A., Giannicchi, A., Shah, Z., Househ, M., Hamdi, M. (2020). Blockchain technologies to mitigate Covid-19 challenges: A scoping review. *Computer Methods and Programs in Biomedicine Update*, (November), 100001. DOI: 10.1016/j.cmpbup.2020.100001.

Benil, T. and Jasper, J. (2020). Cloud based security on outsourcing using Blockchain in E-health systems. *Computer Networks*, 178(June), 107344. DOI: 10.1016/j.comnet.2020.107344.

Chen, L., Lee, W.-K., Chang, C.-C., Choo, K.-K.R., Zhang, N. (2019). Blockchain based searchable encryption for electronic health record sharing. *Future Generation Computer Systems*, 95, 420–429. DOI: 10.1016/j.future.2019.01.018.

Choudhury, T., Khanna, A., Toe, T.T., Khurana, M., Nhu, N.G. (eds) (2021). *Blockchain Applications in IoT Ecosystem*. Springer, Cham.

Dagher, G.G., Mohler, J., Milojkovic, M., Marella, P.B. (2018). Ancile: Privacy-preserving framework for access control and interoperability of electronic health records using Blockchain technology. *Sustainable Cities and Society*, 39(February), 283–297. DOI: 10.1016/j.scs.2018.02.014.

Ferrer-Gomila, J.L., Francisca Hinarejos, M., Isern-Deyà, A.P. (2019). A fair contract signing protocol with blockchain support. *Electronic Commerce Research and Applications*, 36(January), 100869. DOI: 10.1016/j.elerap.2019.100869.

Gul, M.J., Subramanian, B., Paul, A., Kim, J. (2020). Blockchain for public health care in smart society. *Microprocessors and Microsystems*, 103524. DOI: 10.1016/j.micpro.2020.103524.

Huang, H., Zhu, P., Xiao, F., Sun, X., Huang, Q. (2020). A Blockchain-based scheme for privacy-preserving and secure sharing of medical. *Computer & Security*, 99. DOI: 10.1016/j.cose.2020.102010.

Huang, H., Sun, X., Xiao, F., Zhu, P., Wang, W. (2021). Blockchain-based eHealth system for auditable EHRs manipulation in cloud environments. *Journal of Parallel and Distributed Computing*, 148, 46–57. DOI: 10.1016/j.jpdc.2020.10.002.

Hussein, A.F., ArunKumar, N., Ramírez-González, G., Abdulhay, E., Tavares, J.M.R.S., De Albuquerque, V.H.C. (2018). A medical records managing and securing Blockchain based system supported by a genetic algorithm and discrete wavelet transform. *Cognitive Systems Research*, 52, 1–11. DOI: 10.1016/j.cogsys.2018.05.004.

Islam, A. and Young Shin, S. (2020). A Blockchain-based secure healthcare scheme with the assistance of unmanned aerial vehicle in Internet of Things. *Computers and Electrical Engineering*, 84, 106627. DOI: 10.1016/j.compeleceng.2020.106627.

Khanna, A., Sah, A., Choudhury, T. (2020a). Intelligent mobile edge computing: A deep learning based approach. *International Conference on Advances in Computing and Data Sciences*, 107–116. Springer, Singapore. DOI: 10.1007/978-981-15-6634-9_11.

Khanna, A., Sah, A., Choudhury T., Maheshwari, P. (2020b). Blockchain technology for hospitality industry. *European, Mediterranean, and Middle Eastern Conference on Information Systems*, 99–112. DOI: 10.1007/978-3-030-63396-7_7.

Negi, D., Sah, A., Rawat, S., Choudhury, T., Khanna, A. (2021). Block chain platforms and smart contracts. In *Blockchain Applications in IoT Ecosystem*, Choudhury, T., Khanna, A., Toe, T.T., Khurana, M., Nhu, N.G. (eds). Springer, Cham.

Nguyen, D.C., Pathirana, P.N., Ding, M., Seneviratne, A. (2020). Blockchain for 5G and beyond networks: A state of the art survey. *Journal of Network and Computer Applications*, 166, 102693. DOI: 10.1016/j.jnca.2020.102693.

Rawat, S. and Sah, A. (2012). An approach to enhance the software and services of health care centre. *Computer Engineering and Intelligent Systems*, 3(7), 126–137.

Sah, A., Dumka, A., Rawat, S. (2018). Web technology systems integration using SOA and web services. In *Handbook of Research on Contemporary Perspectives on Web-Based Systems*, Elçi, A. (ed.). IGI Global, Hershey, PA [Online]. Available at: https://doi.org/10.4018/978-1-5225-5384-7.ch002.

Tanwar, S., Parekh, K., Evans, R. (2020). Blockchain-based electronic healthcare record system for healthcare 4.0 applications. *Journal of Information Security and Applications*, 50, 102407. DOI: 10.1016/j.jisa.2019.102407.

Tripathi, G., Ahad, M.A., Paiva, S. (2019). A Blockchain based approach for smart healthcare system. *Healthcare*, 8(1), 100391. DOI: 10.1016/j.hjdsi.2019.100391.

Wang, Z., Luo, N., Zhou, P. (2020). GuardHealth: Blockchain empowered secure data management and graph convolutional network enabled anomaly detection in smart healthcare. *Journal of Parallel and Distributed Computing*, 142, 1–12. DOI: 10.1016/j.jpdc.2020.03.004.

4

Analyzing and Modeling the Challenges Faced by the Healthcare Sector in the Adoption Process of Blockchain Technologies

Using Blockchain technology, information can be recorded and shared in a community. This study aims to identify the challenges healthcare organizations face in adopting Blockchain technology to improve patient care. Three hypotheses are being proposed by taking three independent variables and one dependent variable. Target populations are mainly the IT staff working in the hospitals. The respondents were selected from the employees who had IT information about their individual healthcare firms' present and future tasks. A total of 536 questionnaires were sent for a survey, out of which only 350 valid responses are being counted as the rest are mostly unanswered or partially filled. The findings showed that the proposed hypotheses are being accepted. This study will help Blockchain providers and the healthcare industry to understand the problems and find a probable solution. Further analysis can be extended to find a solution to the challenges pointed out in the research.

4.1. Introduction

Blockchain (BC) is one of the latest innovative technologies first introduced in 2009. BC operates by storing data in decentralized recording ledger devices with the BC infrastructure (Beck et al. 2017). The organization's foundation is shared, and it works by having both organization clients (who participate in exchanges) and BC

Chapter written by Subhodeep MUKHERJEE, Manish Mohan BARAL and Venkataiah CHITTIPAKA.

excavators (that work with the businesses in a disseminated record). The document is put away in a decentralized organization of hubs produced by all diggers in the organization using cryptographic cycles (Coita et al. 2019). As it is fabricated using agreement systems, computerized marks and hash chains, the BC record has exceptionally secure capacity abilities (Kshetri 2017). BC offers different administrations like discernibility, trustworthiness, classification and non-disavowal because of these high-level highlights, while putting away all data in a public and decentralized way, using security safeguarding (Rios et al. 2018). Banking, insurance, real estate and government are only a few industries where BC can be used. Various researchers have highlighted the applications of BC in the healthcare industries and how BC can bring revelation in the healthcare sector (Mukherjee et al. 2021a, 2022b).

Additionally, this technology has the potential to benefit health information exchanges (HIEs) (Mazlan et al. 2020; Hussien et al. 2021). However, the technology is not yet fully mature and cannot be used as a panacea in the healthcare industry (McGhin et al. 2019b; Khatri et al. 2021). BC technology allows healthcare stakeholders to share their network access without compromising security or integrity (Saranya and Murugan 2021). Access to public and private keys, proof-of-work and distributed data in cryptography give healthcare information a new level of integrity (Siyal et al. 2019). Drugs can be easily tracked as they move from the manufacturer to the patient using BC technology. They can also be followed more quickly as they move through the supply chain, which helps to prevent drug fraud (Mukherjee et al. 2022).

In terms of revenue and employment, healthcare is now one of India's largest industries. Healthcare encompasses hospitals, doctors, clinical trials, outsourcing, telemedicine, tourism, health insurance and medical equipment. The Indian healthcare industry is growing as the country's population, services and public and private spending all increase (Rout et al. 2019). The Indian healthcare system is divided into two major components: public and private (Mukherjee et al. 2022a). The government provides a small number of secondary and tertiary healthcare institutions in major cities. It is concerned with providing basic healthcare in rural areas through primary healthcare centers (PHCs). The private sector provides most high school, tertiary and quaternary care in metro and level I and level II cities.

IT innovations that link up many islands of healthcare information can improve quality and decrease costs significantly, for instance, by keeping the different providers informed, thus reducing omission or commission errors (Zhang et al. 2018). With the help of this study, healthcare companies can identify the challenges they face when implementing BC in their systems. The literature review identified technical, social and organizational challenges.

The rest of the chapter is designed as follows. Section 4.2 discusses the literature review. Section 4.3 discusses the research methodology. Section 4.4 discusses the data analysis. Section 4.5 highlights the discussion. Section 4.6 gives the conclusion of the study.

4.2. Literature review

4.2.1. *Blockchain in healthcare*

BC technology is a community-based decentralized digital ledger that allows people to record and exchange information (Hathaliya et al. 2019). Third-party intermediaries are replaced as confidence keepers in BC cryptography (Shahnaz et al. 2019). By attempting to decentralize EHRs, this technology will provide a new paradigm for HIE, enhancing device efficiency and protection (Shahnaz et al. 2019). BC is crucial because it instills confidence in peer-to-peer networks. The consensus process, distributed ledger and public-key cryptography are critical components of BC technology (McGhin et al. 2019a; Tanwar et al. 2020). The BC platform uses a decentralized architecture to ensure that all network participants meet the application's requirements.

Exceptional privacy and protection requirements apply in the healthcare sector due to additional regulatory provisions to protect patient medical records. In the Internet period, as distributed storage and the appropriation of versatile well-being gadgets increment the trading of reports and information, so does the danger of vindictive assaults and the danger of private data being undermined as it is traded (Yaqoob et al. 2021). As well-being data turns out to be more open than awesome gadgets and patients visit numerous doctors, the sharing and security of this information are becoming worrisome. Validation, interoperability, information sharing, the exchange of clinical data and contemplations for versatile well-being are a portion of the particular guidelines confronting the medical services industry (Gökalp et al. 2018; Zhang et al. 2018; Khezr et al. 2019). The applications of BC in healthcare are as follows:

– Clinical data sharing: the framework's sharing of clinical information among different elements is essential for BC in medical services. EHRs and EMRs contain profoundly confidential and crucial patient clinical data that should be securely put away, traded, handled and accessed.

– Global data sharing: there are times when patients fly outside of their nation of origin for travel or other reasons. Likewise, there are times that they should look for clinical guidelines for treating an illness (Pirtle and Ehrenfeld 2018; Kassab et al.

2019). Particular specialists/medical clinics in the other nation should know about the patient's medical care subtleties to give better well-being administration.

– Maintaining medical history: the BC innovation can likewise store and save a patient's clinical history (Pandey and Litoriya 2020; Yaqoob et al. 2021). Patients can go to incoherent clinics, for instance, and the general chain of their clinical history may not be open or kept up (due to irregularity and inaccessibility of records).

– Healthcare data access control: clients' control/hold over their information is disintegrating because of ongoing innovative progressions (Shah et al. 2018; Onik et al. 2019). Clients are frequently ignorant of the offices that approach their clinical knowledge, for what reasons, and whether they can do so. This is particularly valid for medical services information.

– Drug supply chain management: clinical medication supply on the board is essential in the present clinical industry, yet intricacies and misfortunes likewise assail it because of forgers and pilferers. BC will keep up the detectability of such production network tasks and improve the general interaction's believability (Hussien et al. 2019; Yaqoob et al. 2021).

4.3. Challenges of Blockchain in healthcare

4.3.1. *Technical challenges (TC)*

"Technical difficulties" refer to hardware and software problems with the information technology infrastructure. The scalability problem with BC technology was due to the network's low rate of handling transactions per second. Authorization and protection problems, high energy usage and low processing charges are two of the more technological challenges found (Dutta et al. 2020; Kumar and Krishnamoorthy 2020; Alazab et al. 2021; Mikalef et al. 2021).

H1: TC influences BCH.

4.3.2. *Social challenges (SC)*

Firms face various social problems, the most common of which is regulation. The BC regulatory framework varies from country to country. Despite legitimate privacy concerns, it is difficult for legal authorities to grant access to medical records due to decentralized medical data and the absence of an intermediary

(Francisco and Swanson 2018; Verhoeven et al. 2018; Di Vaio and Varriale 2020; Koh et al. 2020; Orji et al. 2020). BC implementation of healthcare may be hampered by a lack of government legislation and guidelines.

H2: SC influences BCH.

4.3.3. *Organizational challenges (OC)*

In most organizations, there are setup and exchange costs, interoperability issues and technical skills shortages that must be addressed to succeed. The absence of certainty among parties and confined open principles has been reprimanded for the interoperability issue, making a substantial trade of well-being data between medical services associations troublesome (Clohessy et al. 2019; Kamble et al. 2019; Queiroz and Fosso Wamba 2019; Sheel and Nath 2019; Gökalp et al. 2020; Wamba and Queiroz 2020; Kouhizadeh et al. 2021). Fundamental mechanical abilities and IT experts who are specialists in working on the innovation are expected to keep an incorporated drug inventory network between BC partners. While BC sets aside cash for the long haul, the underlying expense of establishment is high.

H3: OC influences BCH.

4.4. Research methodology

Primary and secondary data collection methods are employed. To collect preliminary data, the target population is surveyed using questionnaires (Mukherjee et al. 2021). The secondary data collection method consists of articles published in journals, magazines, reports, etc. (Mukherjee et al. 2021b). It is necessary to prepare a structured questionnaire to conduct survey-based research. This campaign is aimed at hospital employees familiar with BC's technology and know-how to use it. For this study, simple random sampling was used as a sampling technique (Baral and Verma 2021). The questionnaire was sent to 536 selected respondents, out of which 350 respondents returned the filled questionnaires, which were appropriately and correctly filled in. After collection of the common method, the collected data was checked for bias (Mukherjee and Chittipaka 2021). For this, the Harman test was performed, giving 33.451%, which was below the threshold level of 50% (Mukherjee et al. 2022b). Using exploratory factor analysis (EFA), confirmatory factor analysis (CFA) and structural equation modeling (SEM), further data analysis is performed.

Item Gender	Frequency	Percentage
Male	226	64.57
Female	124	35.43
Years of experience using online services		
< 3 years	142	40.57
3–5 years	81	23.14
> 5 years	127	36.29

Table 4.1. *Respondents' demographics. Source: output obtained from survey data*

4.5. Data analysis

CA, or Cronbach's alpha, measures the reliability and validity of the data. The recommended values should be greater than 0.70 (Kline 1999). CA values for the TC variable are 0.951; CA values for the SC variable are 0.849; CA values for the OC variable are 0.843. EFA is calculated to group the variables in some constructs. To check the correlation between the factors, Bartlett's test of sphericity is performed (Moss and Hendry 2002). The principal axis factoring and varimax rotation method are followed for EFA (Mukherjee et al. 2022a).

Kaiser–Meyer–Olkin measure of sampling adequacy		.866
Bartlett's test of sphericity	Approx. Chi-square	3314.042
	Df	91
	Sig.	.000

Table 4.2. *KMO and Bartlett's test. Source: output obtained from SPSS 20.0. Authors' results*

The eigenvalues should be greater than one, which was extracted for maximum variance explained (Tabachnick et al. 2007). Total variance (TVE) extracted for the three components are 36.511%, 20.066% and 15.763. The cumulative frequency for the TVE is 72.340%. The rotated components matrix is shown in Table 4.3. All of the indicators are grouped into three constructs (Mukherjee et al. 2022c).

	Rotated component matrix		
	Component		
	1	2	3
TC1	.854		
TC2	.920		
TC3	.923		
TC4	.886		
TC5	.896		
SC1		.865	
SC2		.819	
SC3		.828	
SC4		.889	
SC5		.494	
OC1			.794
OC2			.836
OC3			.790
OC4			.853

Table 4.3. *Rotated factor matrix. Source: output obtained from SPSS 20.0. Authors' results*

CFA is performed to check the convergent and divergent validity (Nunnally 1978). Three constructs, along with their indicators, are shown in Figure 4.1.

Goodness-of-fit indices	Default model	Benchmark
Absolute goodness-of-fit measure		
$\chi 2$/df (CMIN/DF)	1.848	Lower Limit:1.0 Upper Limit 2.0/3.0 or 5.0
GFI	0.948	>0.90
Incremental fit measure		
CFI	0.981	⩾0.90
IFI	0.981	⩾0.90
TLI	0.976	⩾0.90
Parsimony fit measure		
PCFI	0.798	⩾0.50
PNFI	0.780	⩾0.50

Table 4.4. *Model fit measures for the confirmatory factor analysis. Source: output obtained from AMOS 22.0. Authors' results*

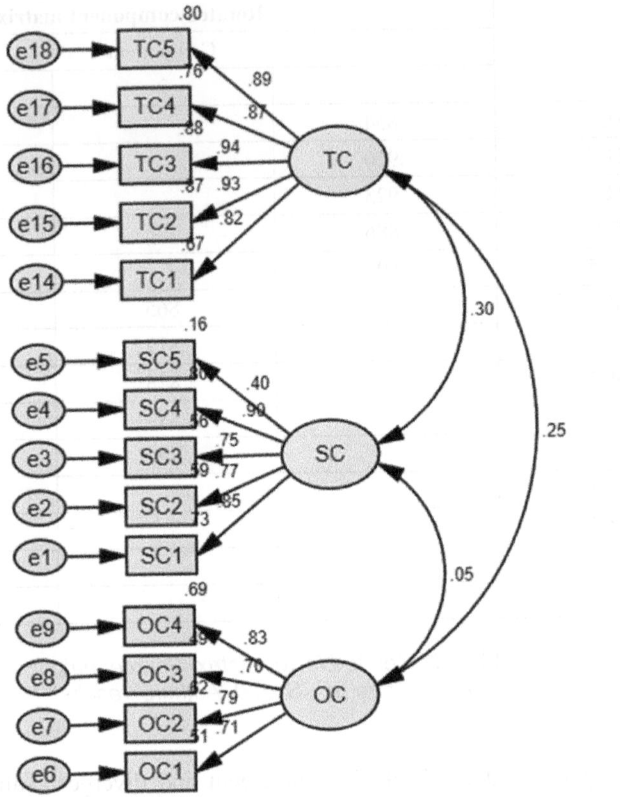

Figure 4.1. *Confirmatory factor analysis for the latent variables. Source: output obtained from AMOS 22.0. Authors' results*

The average variance extracted (AVE) for the values is shown in Table 4.5.

	AVE	Variance extracted between factors		
		TC	SC	OC
TC	0.911	1		
SC	0.785	0.723	1	
OC	0.823	0.754	0.754	1

Table 4.5. *Construct correlation and AVE. Source: output obtained from AMOS 22.0. Authors' results*

	Estimate	SE.	CR.	P
SC1<---SC	0.852			
SC2<---SC	0.769	0.056	13.73	0.000
SC3<---SC	0.751	0.054	13.90	0.000
SC4<---SC	0.895	0.053	16.88	0.000
SC5<---SC	0.399	0.068	5.86	0.000
OC1<---OC	0.711			
OC2<---OC	0.787	0.088	8.94	0.000
OC3<---OC	0.701	0.086	8.15	0.000
OC4<---OC	0.828	0.089	9.30	0.000
TC1<---TC	0.821			
TC2<---TC	0.930	0.055	16.91	0.000
TC3<---TC	0.937	0.056	16.73	0.000
TC4<---TC	0.874	0.056	15.61	0.000
TC5<---TC	0.892	0.055	15.78	0.000

Table 4.6. *Path analysis result for confirmatory factor analysis. Source: output obtained from AMOS 22.0. Authors' results*

Goodness-of-fit indices	Default model	Benchmark
Absolute goodness-of-fit measure		
CMIN/Df	1.551	⩽3
Absolute badness-of-fit measure		
RMSEA	0.040	⩽0.08
Incremental fit measure		
CFI	0.982	⩾0.90
IFI	0.982	⩾0.90
TLI	0.979	⩾0.90
Parsimony fit measure		
PCFI	0.828	⩾0.50
PNFI	0.803	⩾0.50

Table 4.7. *Model parameter for the structural model. Source: output obtained from AMOS 22.0. Authors' results*

Table 4.6 shows the path analysis result for the CFA model. The P-value for the indicators is 0.000, so they satisfy the measurements items (Baral et al. 2022). Figure 4.2 shows the final model. TC: Technological challenges have five indicators TC1, TC2, TC3, TC4 and TC5; OC: Organizational challenges have five indicators OC1, OC2, OC3, OC4 and OC5; SC: Social challenges have four indicators SC1, SC2, SC3 and SC4 (Mukherjee et al. 2021). Table 4.7 shows the model fit measures for the SEM model.

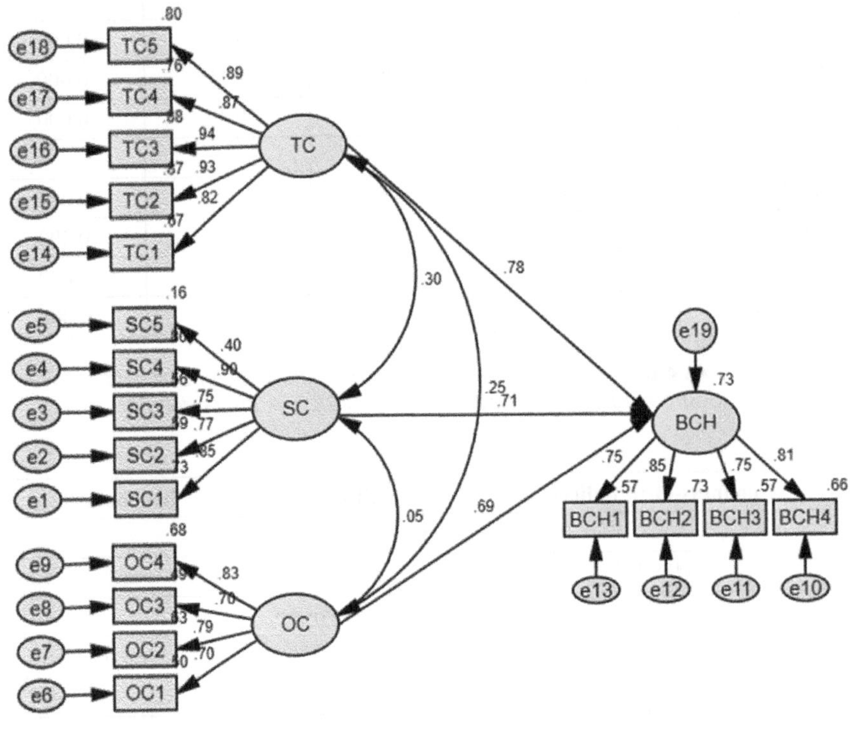

Figure 4.2. *The final model. Source: output obtained from AMOS 22.0. Authors' results*

	Estimate	SE.	CR.	P	Hypothesis
BCH <---TC	.78	.062	12.58	.000	Accepted
BCH <---SC	.71	.054	13.15	.000	Accepted
BCH<---OC	.61	.078	7.82	.000	Accepted

Table 4.8. *Structural model results. Source: output obtained from AMOS 22.0. Authors' results*

4.6. Discussion

Worldwide, healthcare systems are under tremendous stress due to the pandemic, which has resulted in supply chain disruptions, counterfeit medical products, health data management and security, among other issues. New and emerging technologies, such as Blockchain, the technology behind cryptocurrencies, can address these issues (Saranya and Murugan 2021). This study will identify the challenges that healthcare sectors will face in implementing a BC system. The three challenges identified are mainly the technical challenges, social challenges and organizational challenges. TC stands for technical challenges faced by the BC adopters. These challenges have been identified in previous studies (Sadhya and Sadhya 2018; Onik et al. 2019; Pandey and Litoriya 2020; Saranya and Murugan 2021). SC stands for the social challenges faced by the BC adopters. These challenges and results have been identified in previous studies (Shah et al. 2018; Shahnaz et al. 2019; Siyal et al. 2019; Wamba and Queiroz 2020; Wong et al. 2020). OC stands for organizational challenges faced by the BC adopters. These challenges and results have been identified in previous studies (Zhang et al. 2018; Zhao et al. 2019; Wong et al. 2020; Yaqoob et al. 2021). Blockchain adoption in healthcare faces several challenges, including technical issues and ownership concerns (Kant Pal et al. 2021). Technological challenges such as processing speed and massive data duplication will be resolved as technology develops (Zhang et al. 2018). As a result of its benefits in payment integrity, data interoperability and security, Blockchain can transform the healthcare ecosystem. A time-consuming and labor-intensive pharmaceutical research process, for example, would be transformed into a more efficient, data-driven one (Tanwar et al. 2020). Assigning patient control, ownership and access to patient data using a Blockchain solution would make this possible.

4.7. Conclusion

As part of the study, healthcare companies will be asked to describe their challenges when implementing BC in their systems. Many industrial sectors use BC to improve transparency and tracking. After completing a structured literature review, a list of issues facing healthcare organizations was compiled for the research project. An Indian hospital is currently working on a survey-based research questionnaire. For data analysis and modeling, exploratory factor analysis and structural equation modeling are used. As a result, more challenges can be identified by extending this study into other fields.

4.8. References

Alazab, M., Alhyari, S., Awajan, A., Abdallah, A.B. (2021). Blockchain technology in supply chain management: An empirical study of the factors affecting user adoption/acceptance. *Cluster Computing*, 24(1), 83–101. DOI: 10.1007/s10586-020-03200-4.

Baral, M.M. and Verma, A. (2021). Cloud computing adoption for healthcare: An empirical study using SEM approach. *FIIB Business Review*, 10(3), 255–275. DOI: 10.1177/231971 45211012505.

Baral, M.M., Mukherjee, S., Nagariya, R., Singh Patel, B., Pathak, A., Chittipaka, V. (2022). Analysis of factors impacting firm performance of MSMEs: Lessons learnt from COVID-19. *Benchmarking: An International Journal*, (ahead-of-print). DOI: 10.1108/ BIJ-11-2021-0660.

Beck, R., Avital, M., Rossi, M., Thatcher, J.B. (2017). Blockchain technology in business and information systems research. *Business & Information Systems Engineering*, 59(6), 381–384. DOI: 10.1007/s12599-017-0505-1.

Clohessy, T., Acton, T., Rogers, N. (2019). Blockchain adoption: Technological, organisational and environmental considerations. *Business Transformation through Blockchain*, 47–76. DOI: 10.1007/978-3-319-98911-2_2.

Coita, D.C., Abrudan, M.M., Matei, M.C. (2019). Effects of the blockchain technology on human resources and marketing: An exploratory study. In *Strategic Innovative Marketing and Tourism*, Kavoura, A., Kefallonitis, E., Giovanis, A. (eds). Springer, Cham. DOI: 10.1007/978-3-030-12453-3_79.

Di Vaio, A. and Varriale, L. (2020). Blockchain technology in supply chain management for sustainable performance: Evidence from the airport industry. *International Journal of Information Management*, 52(March), 0–1. DOI: 10.1016/j.ijinfomgt.2019.09.010.

Dutta, P., Choi, T.M., Somani, S., Butala, R. (2020). Blockchain technology in supply chain operations: Applications, challenges and research opportunities. *Transportation Research Part E: Logistics and Transportation Review*, 142, 102067. DOI: 10.1016/J.TRE.2020. 102067.

Francisco, K. and Swanson, D. (2018). The supply chain has no clothes: Technology adoption of blockchain for supply chain transparency. *Logistics*, 2(1), 2. DOI: 10.3390/logistics 2010002.

Gökalp, E., Gökalp, M.O., Çoban, S., Eren, P.E. (2018). Analysing opportunities and challenges of integrated blockchain technologies in healthcare. *Lecture Notes in Business Information Processing*, 333, 174–183. DOI: 10.1007/978-3-030-00060-8_13.

Gökalp, E., Gökalp, M.O., Çoban, S. (2020). Blockchain-based supply chain management: Understanding the determinants of adoption in the context of organizations. *Information Systems Management*, 39(3), 1–22. DOI: 10.1080/10580530.2020.1812014.

Hathaliya, J., Sharma, P., Tanwar, S., Gupta, R. (2019). Blockchain-based remote patient monitoring in healthcare 4.0. *Proceedings of the 2019 IEEE 9th International Conference on Advanced Computing, IACC 2019*, 87–91. DOI: 10.1109/IACC48062.2019.8971593.

Hussien, H.M., Yasin, S.M., Udzir, S.N.I., Zaidan, A.A., Zaidan, B.B. (2019). A systematic review for enabling of develop a Blockchain technology in healthcare applications: Taxonomy, substantially analysis, motivations, challenges, recommendations and future direction. *Journal of Medical Systems*, 43(10). DOI: 10.1007/s10916-019-1445-8.

Hussien, H.M., Yasin, S.M., Udzir, N.I., Ninggal, M.I.H., Salman, S. (2021). Blockchain technology in the healthcare industry: Trends and opportunities. *Journal of Industrial Information Integration*, 22, 100217. DOI: 10.1016/J.JII.2021.100217.

Kamble, S., Gunasekaran, A., Arha, H. (2019). Understanding the Blockchain technology adoption in supply chains – Indian context. *International Journal of Production Research*, 57(7), 2009–2033. DOI: 10.1080/00207543.2018.1518610.

Kant Pal, S., Mukherjee, S., Baral, M.M., Aggarwal, S. (2021). Problems of big data adoption in the healthcare industries. *Asia Pacific Journal of Health Management*, 16(4), 282–287. DOI: 10.24083/apjhm.v16i4.1359.

Kassab, M.H., DeFranco, J., Malas, T., Laplante, P., Destefanis, G., Graciano Neto, V.V. (2019). Exploring research in Blockchain for healthcare and a roadmap for the future. *IEEE Transactions on Emerging Topics in Computing*. DOI: 10.1109/TETC.2019.2936881.

Khatri, S., Alzahrani, F.A., Ansari, M.T.J., Agrawal, A., Kumar, R., Khan, R.A. (2021). A systematic analysis on Blockchain integration with healthcare domain: Scope and challenges. *IEEE Access*, 9, 84666–84687. DOI: 10.1109/ACCESS.2021.3087608.

Khezr, S., Moniruzzaman, M., Yassine, A., Benlamri, R. (2019). Blockchain technology in healthcare: A comprehensive review and directions for future research. *Applied Sciences (Switzerland)*, 9(9). DOI: 10.3390/app9091736.

Kline, R.B. (1999). Book review: Psychometric theory (3rd ed.). *Journal of Psychoeducational Assessment*, 17(3), 275–280 DOI: 10.1177/073428299901700307.

Koh, L., Dolgui, A., Sarkis, J. (2020). Blockchain in transport and logistics – Paradigms and transitions. *International Journal of Production Research*, 58(7), 2054–2062. DOI: 10.1080/00207543.2020.1736428.

Kouhizadeh, M., Saberi, S., Sarkis, J. (2021). Blockchain technology and the sustainable supply chain: Theoretically exploring adoption barriers. *International Journal of Production Economics*, 231, 107831. DOI: 10.1016/j.ijpe.2020.107831.

Kshetri, N. (2017). Blockchain's roles in strengthening cybersecurity and protecting privacy. *Telecommunications Policy*, 41(10), 1027–1038. DOI: 10.1016/j.telpol.2017.09.003.

Kumar, A. and Krishnamoorthy, B. (2020). Business analytics adoption in firms: A qualitative study elaborating TOE framework in India. *International Journal of Global Business and Competitiveness*, 15(2), 80–93. DOI: 10.1007/s42943-020-00013-5.

Mazlan, A.A., Daud, S.M., Sam, S.M., Abas, H., Rasid, S.Z.A., Yusof, M.F. (2020). Scalability challenges in healthcare Blockchain system – A systematic review. *IEEE Access*, 8, 23663–23673. DOI: 10.1109/ACCESS.2020.2969230.

McGhin, T., Choo, K.K.R., Liu, C.Z., He, D. (2019). Blockchain in healthcare applications: Research challenges and opportunities. *Journal of Network and Computer Applications*, 135(September 2018), 62–75. DOI: 10.1016/j.jnca.2019.02.027.

Mikalef, P., Lemmer, K., Schaefer, C., Ylinen, M., Fjørtoft, S.O., Torvatn, H.Y., Gupta, M., Niehaves, B. (2021). Enabling AI capabilities in government agencies: A study of determinants for European municipalities. *Government Information Quarterly*, 101596. DOI: 10.1016/j.giq.2021.101596.

Moss, J. and Hendry, G. (2002). Use of electronic surveys in course evaluation. *British Journal of Educational Technology*, 33(5), 583–592. DOI: 10.1111/1467-8535.00293.

Mukherjee, S. and Chittipaka, V. (2021). Analysing the adoption of intelligent agent technology in food supply chain management: An empirical evidence. *FIIB Business Review*, 231971452110592. DOI: 10.1177/23197145211059243.

Mukherjee, S., Baral, M.M., Venkataiah, C., Pal, S.K., Nagariya, R. (2021a). Service robots are an option for contactless services due to the COVID-19 pandemic in the hotels. *Decision*, 48(4), 445–460. DOI: 10.1007/s40622-021-00300-x.

Mukherjee, S., Chittipaka, V., Baral, M.M. (2021b). Developing a model to highlight the relation of digital trust with privacy and security for the Blockchain technology. In *Blockchain Technology and Applications for Digital Marketing*, Bansal, R., Malyadri, P., Singh, A., Pervez, A. (eds). IGI Global, Hershey, PA. DOI: 10.4018/978-1-7998-8081-3.ch007.

Mukherjee, S., Mohan Baral, M., Srivastava, S.C., Jana, B. (2021c). Analyzing the problems faced by fashion retail stores due to Covid-19 outbreak. *Parikalpana-KIIT Journal of Management*, 17(I). DOI: 10.23862/kiit-parikalpana/2021/v17/i1/209031.

Mukherjee, S., Baral, M.M., Chittipaka, V. (2022a). How to improve organizational performance using big data in the hotels. In *Integrating Blockchain Technology Into the Circular Economy*, Khan, S.A.R. (ed.). IGI Global, Hershey, PA. DOI: 10.4018/978-1-7998-7642-7.ch002.

Mukherjee, S., Baral, M.M., Chittipaka, V. (2022b). Studying the adoption of blockchain technology in the manufacturing firms. In *Utilizing Blockchain Technologies in Manufacturing and Logistics Management*, Goyal, S.B., Praddep, N., Shukla, P.K., Ghonge, M.M., Ravi, R.V. (eds). IGI Global, Hershey, PA. DOI: 10.4018/978-1-7998-8697-6.ch004.

Mukherjee, S., Baral, M.M., Chittipaka, V., Pal, S.K., Nagariya, R. (2022c). Investigating sustainable development for the COVID-19 vaccine supply chain: A structural equation modelling approach. *Journal of Humanitarian Logistics and Supply Chain Management* (ahead-of-print). DOI: 10.1108/JHLSCM-08-2021-0079.

Mukherjee, S., Chittipaka, V., Baral, M.M. (2022d). Addressing and modeling the challenges faced in the implementation of Blockchain technology in the food and agriculture supply chain. In *Blockchain Technologies and Applications for Digital Governance*, Nijalingappa, P. and Ghonge, M.M. (eds). IGI Global, Hershey, PA. DOI: 10.4018/978-1-7998-8493-4.ch007.

Mukherjee, S., Venkataiah, C., Baral, M.M., Pal, S.K. (2022e). Analyzing the factors that will impact the supply chain of the COVID-19 vaccine: A structural equation modeling approach. *Journal of Statistics and Management Systems*, 1–16. DOI: 10.1080/09720510.2021.1966955.

Nunnally, J.C. (1978). An overview of psychological measurement. In *Clinical Diagnosis of Mental Disorders*, Wolman, B.B. (ed.). Springer, New York.

Onik, Md. M.H., Aich, S., Yang, J., Kim, C.-S., Kim, H.-C. (2019). Blockchain in healthcare: challenges and solutions. In *Big Data Analytics for Intelligent Healthcare Management*, Dey, N. (ed.). Elsevier, London. DOI: 10.1016/b978-0-12-818146-1.00008-8.

Orji, I.J., Kusi-Sarpong, S., Huang, S., Vazquez-Brust, D. (2020). Evaluating the factors that influence Blockchain adoption in the freight logistics industry. *Transportation Research Part E: Logistics and Transportation Review*, 141, 102025. DOI: 10.1016/j.tre.2020.102025.

Pandey, P. and Litoriya, R. (2020). Implementing healthcare services on a large scale: Challenges and remedies based on blockchain technology. *Health Policy and Technology*, 9(1), 69–78. DOI: 10.1016/j.hlpt.2020.01.004.

Pirtle, C. and Ehrenfeld, J. (2018). Blockchain for healthcare: The next generation of medical records? *Journal of Medical Systems*, 42(9), 1–3, Springer, New York. DOI: 10.1007/s10916-018-1025-3.

Queiroz, M.M. and Fosso Wamba, S. (2019). Blockchain adoption challenges in supply chain: An empirical investigation of the main drivers in India and the USA. *International Journal of Information Management*, 46, 70–82. DOI: 10.1016/j.ijinfomgt.2018.11.021.

Rios, R., Fernandez-Gago, C., Lopez, J. (2018). Modelling privacy-aware trust negotiations. *Computers and Security*, 77, 773–789. DOI: 10.1016/j.cose.2017.09.015.

Rout, S.K., Sahu, K.S., Mahapatra, S. (2019). Utilization of health care services in public and private healthcare in India: Causes and determinants. *International Journal of Healthcare Management*, 14(2), 509–516. DOI: 10.1080/20479700.2019.1665882.

Sadhya, V. and Sadhya, H. (2018). Barriers to adoption of Blockchain technology. *Proceedings of the 24th Americas Conference on Information Systems*, 1–10.

Saranya, R. and Murugan, A. (2021). A systematic review of enabling Blockchain in healthcare system: Analysis, current status, challenges and future direction. *Materials Today: Proceedings*. DOI: 10.1016/J.MATPR.2021.07.105.

Shah, B., Shah, N., Shakhla, S., Sawant, V. (2018). Remodeling the healthcare industry by employing Blockchain technology. *2018 International Conference on Circuits and Systems in Digital Enterprise Technology, ICCSDET 2018*. DOI: 10.1109/ICCSDET.2018.8821113.

Shahnaz, A., Qamar, U., Khalid, A. (2019). Using Blockchain for electronic health records. *IEEE Access*, 7, 147782–147795. DOI: 10.1109/ACCESS.2019.2946373.

Sheel, A. and Nath, V. (2019). Effect of blockchain technology adoption on supply chain adaptability, agility, alignment and performance. *Management Research Review*, 42(12), 1353–1374. DOI: 10.1108/MRR-12-2018-0490.

Siyal, A.A., Junejo, A.Z., Zawish, M., Ahmed, K., Khalil, A., Soursou, G. (2019). Applications of Blockchain technology in medicine and healthcare: Challenges and future perspectives. *Cryptography 2019*, 3(1), 3. DOI: 10.3390/CRYPTOGRAPHY3010003.

Tabachnick, B.G., Fidell, L.S., Ullman, J.B. (2007). *Using Multivariate Statistics*, 5th edition. Pearson, Boston, MA.

Tanwar, S., Parekh, K., Evans, R. (2020). Blockchain-based electronic healthcare record system for healthcare 4.0 applications. *Journal of Information Security and Applications*, 50, 102407. DOI: 10.1016/j.jisa.2019.102407.

Verhoeven, P., Sinn, F., Herden, T.T. (2018). Examples from Blockchain implementations in logistics and supply chain management: Exploring the mindful use of a new technology. *Logistics 2018*, 2(3), 20. DOI: 10.3390/LOGISTICS2030020.

Wamba, S.F. and Queiroz, M.M. (2020). Blockchain in the operations and supply chain management: Benefits, challenges and future research opportunities. *International Journal of Information Management*, 52, 102064, Elsevier. DOI: 10.1016/j.ijinfomgt.2019.102064.

Wong, L.W., Leong, L.Y., Hew, J.J., Tan, G.W.H., Ooi, K.B. (2020). Time to seize the digital evolution: Adoption of blockchain in operations and supply chain management among Malaysian SMEs. *International Journal of Information Management*, 52, 101997. DOI: 10.1016/j.ijinfomgt.2019.08.005.

Yaqoob, I., Salah, K., Jayaraman, R., Al-Hammadi, Y. (2021). Blockchain for healthcare data management: Opportunities, challenges, and future recommendations. In *Neural Computing and Applications*, MacIntyre, J. (ed.). Springer Science and Business Media Deutschland GmbH. DOI: 10.1007/s00521-020-05519-w.

Zhang, P., Schmidt, D.C., White, J., Lenz, G. (2018). Blockchain technology use cases in healthcare. *Advances in Computers*, 111, 1–41. DOI: 10.1016/bs.adcom.2018.03.006.

Zhao, G., Liu, S., Lopez, C., Lu, H., Elgueta, S., Chen, H., Boshkoska, B.M. (2019). Blockchain technology in agri-food value chain management: A synthesis of applications, challenges and future research directions. *Computers in Industry*, 109, 83–99. DOI: 10.1016/j.compind.2019.04.002.

5

Blockchain as an Effective Technology in Maintaining Electronic Health Record Systems

Blockchain technology is one of the most important innovations in the professional world today. It is a distributed network that is made up of an organized list of nodes and connections, with nodes responsible for storing information and chains connecting them. It is the chain of blocks that constitutes the data and helps in maintaining a trust among the individuals. The Blockchain technology is moving on the path of constant change and revolution. The increased use of Blockchain technologies in recent years has compelled experts and academicians to find innovative approaches to implement Blockchain in various fields. Healthcare is the sector that has seen the most growth in terms of data and sales. Security has become increasingly important as the number of electronic health records (EHRs) grows. There has been a push to use Blockchain technologies to make EHRs safer. The increase in the usage of Blockchain technology provides many new application opportunities that include the area of healthcare. EHRs are the most promising use of Blockchains. It can be defined as the health information of the patients that are stored digitally over the network. Blockchain technology has the potential to revolutionize healthcare by putting the user at the center of the clinical system and improving health information transparency, privacy and confidentiality. This chapter not only covers the introduction to Blockchain technology and its background concepts, but it also covers the importance of Blockchain in the healthcare sector. The model for EHR on the basis Blockchain is also proposed. This chapter concludes with the various research challenges in the domain of Blockchain along with a case study.

5.1. Introduction

One of the most precious resources is data. With cyber criminals becoming more skilled at stealing sensitive data, cybersecurity has become one of the most pressing

---

Chapter written by Avita KATAL, Vitesh SETHI, Hussain Falih MAHDI and Tanupriya CHOUDHURY.

global challenges, necessitating cyber protection. Various methods have been suggested in the past to meet the security needs of various organizations, but security attacks have no limits, resulting in the techniques being either compromised or rendered useless. Blockchain technology is the most recent solution to safeguard useful records. It is described as a distributed ledger that holds an ordered list of various items connected by connections known as chains (Katal et al. 2021b). The content included in these blocks, which relate to financial operations, is only accessible to subscribers. An intricate chain of self-managed encryption keys maintains user approval: each authorized user gives a time-sensitive secret identifier that autoblocks it if the decryption timer runs out (Zhang et al. 2018). Blockchain is a modern platform that allows for more autonomous computing. It is based on the principle of public ledger, which acts as an archive for previous transactions surrounding these agents. It is regularly audited by groups of agents (selection is done according to different policies based on the software domain) who audit it on a regular basis. The results of each audit are saved in a block and presented to the entire network. In a cryptographically linked row, blocks are sequentially added to the ledger. Blockchain technology allows data to be shared while maintaining confidentiality. The following are a few of the reasons why Blockchain technology is so common and is being used in various domains:

– When opposed to conventional banks that work on operating hours and rules, Blockchain technology allows for faster transaction settlements. On the contrary, it has no such limitations. It allows for quicker contract settlements.

– Since Blockchain stores data and prevents it from being corrupted, it removes human error. Accuracy is ensured when records are checked as they move from one node to the next.

– Data objectivity is a product of Blockchain technologies. It not only guarantees data confidentiality but also warns users against any data change. If an organization's data is hacked, it cannot be exploited, ensuring a balance between confidentiality and governance.

– In the event that anomalies are discovered, they can still be traced back to their source, which simplifies inquiries and the execution of necessary acts. As a result, quality assurance is achieved.

5.2. Background concepts on Blockchain technology

5.2.1. *Consensus algorithms*

Consensus algorithms are essential components of Blockchain technology which contribute to the creation of a tamper-proof network. It only accepts one source of truth, which is agreed upon by all network members. This technology relies on node-to-node consensus processes to validate data, eliminating the need for intermediaries. Any of the nodes in this network should reach an agreement on the current version of the Blockchain. This increases the system's reliability by making it more complex for the hacker to generate a sudo block and inject it into the distributed network.

Blockchain consensus algorithms are divided into two types: proof-based consensus algorithms and voting-based consensus algorithms (Katal et al. 2021a).

5.2.1.1. *Proof-based consensus algorithms*

The basic idea of evidence-based consensus algorithms says that the node with the greatest proof prevails among numerous nodes joining the network and is given approval in the network to add a new node and get the payment. Many varieties of proof-based consensus algorithms have been applied, including those based on Proof of Work (PoW), Proof of Stake (PoS) or a mixture of the two, as well as a variety of different versions.

5.2.1.2. *Voting-based consensus algorithms*

In order to execute the voting-based consensus algorithm, the nodes within the checking network must be customizable. This allows them to exchange messages more easily. This is the most significant distinction from proof-based consensus algorithms, in which nodes are often able to enter and leave the verifying network. Furthermore, with a voting-based consensus mechanism, all nodes in the network must approve the operations or blocks at the same time, in contrast to maintaining the ledger. They will consult with others before determining whether or not to add their suggested blocks to their chain. Using voting-based consensus algorithms is somewhat close to using standard distributed system fault tolerance methods (Andreev et al. 2018). As a result, voting-based consensus should be built to withstand the following scenarios where any nodes have failed or any nodes have been subverted as well as crashed.

5.2.2. *Types of Blockchain*

The two basic types of Blockchains are private and public Blockchains. Nevertheless, there are various variations, including consortium and hybrid Blockchains. Every Blockchain is made up of nodes that are linked together via a peer-to-peer (P2P) mechanism. Each system node has an up-to-date version of the shared ledger. Each node may confirm operations, transmit and receive data and construct blocks. Firstly, the user initiates the transaction in the network. When the transaction is initiated, the process for the creation of blocks starts which includes the previous block's hash, ownership and the modification history. A nonce creates the cryptographic hash when the first block of a chain is created. The content in the blocks is encrypted until it is mined and is inextricably tied to the nonce and hash. When a block is formed, it is sent to all of the platform's peers for approval. Miners use complex algorithms to solve the extremely difficult mathematical problem of producing an approved hash using a nonce. Because the nonce is only 32 bits long and the hash is 256 bits long, there are roughly 4 billion nonce-hash permutations to mine before finding the proper one. Miners are believed to have uncovered the "golden nonce" when this happens, and the block is included in the chain. When a block is mined correctly, the update is authorized by all servers on the platform, and the miner is rewarded economically. Following acceptance, a current chain is modified with the newly created block. After being added to the chain, the update is disseminated around the system and the action is completed. Figure 5.1 depicts the detailed flow of transaction in the Blockchain.

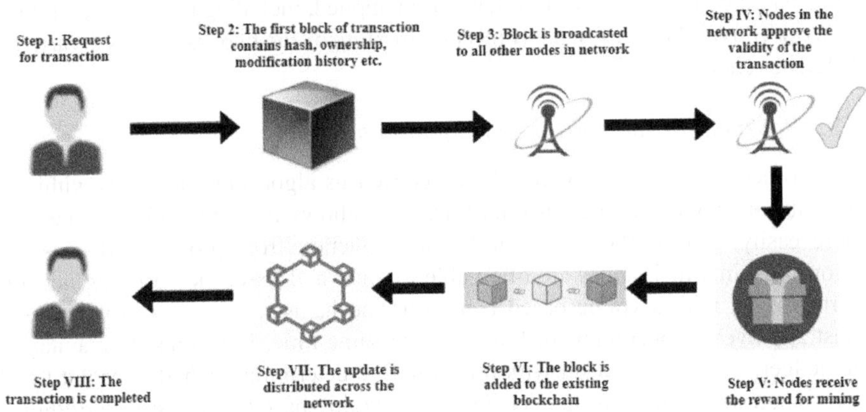

Figure 5.1. *Detailed flow of transaction in the Blockchain. For a color version this figure, see www.iste.co.uk/choudhury/blockchain.zip*

Public Blockchain: it is a distributed ledger scheme with no permissions. Everyone who has an Internet connectivity can join the Blockchain network. A user (also known as a node) who is a member of the public Blockchain is allowed to get the data, validate transactions and mine for the next block. The sharing of cryptocurrency is one of the most popular applications of shared Blockchains. The majority of the time, public Blockchain is safe, if users adhere to safety protocols. However, if consumers do not adhere to the security protocols, it can be dangerous. Bitcoin, Ethereum and Litecoin are some of the most well-known examples (Andreev et al. 2018; Aggarwal et al. 2019).

Private Blockchain: it is a permissioned Blockchain that can only be used within a closed network. Mostly, they are used inside an association or business where only a few people are involved. Protection, authorizations and usability are only a few of the essential resources that are under the jurisdiction of a governing entity. Any basic operations (such as polling, supply chain management and asset ownership) may be performed using a private Blockchain. Multichain and Hyperledger projects are the examples of private Blockchains (i.e. fabric and sawtooth) (Aggarwal et al. 2019).

Consortium Blockchain: it is a somewhat decentralized Blockchain network operated by a number of entities. This sort of Blockchain enables several organizations to collaborate and serve as the regulator for mining and knowledge exchange. Energy Web Foundation and R3 are two examples of this kind of Blockchain (Aggarwal et al. 2019).

Hybrid Blockchain: it is a hybrid Blockchain network that incorporates private and public Blockchain platforms. In this case, the functionality of all Blockchains is used. Subscribers on the hybrid network may keep records about who has access to which Blockchain information. Just a few of the Blockchain's selected documents are allowed to be made available, while the others are kept private in the private network. Users should, however, publish this on the public Blockchain for authentication. Public Blockchains enhance hashing and include additional nodes in the validation process. This improves the Blockchain network's visibility and trust. The hybrid Blockchain "Dragonchain" is an example (Aggarwal et al. 2019).

5.2.3. *Smart contracts*

Szabo coined the word "smart contract" in the mid-1990s, defining it as "a collection of guarantees, defined in electronic format, including rules under which the parties deliver on trust" (Jani 2020). It is a part of Blockchain-based software that helps to enable, implement and monitor contractual arrangements. Its primary objective is to carry out the provisions of an agreement as soon as possible unless certain criteria are satisfied. As a result, smart contracts provide lower settlement costs than conventional schemes, which count on a trustworthy third party to implement and process the terms of a contract. In the literature, several common meanings of a smart contract have been explored. Code that is registered, checked and implemented on a Blockchain is what smart contract code refers to. Smart legal contracts will almost certainly be a hybrid between smart contract code and conventional legal vocabulary. Consider the case of a product seller who enters into a smart legal deal with a manufacturer. The payment terms should be written in code and executed immediately when the product is delivered. However, the manufacturer is likely to insist on an indemnity clause in the deal, in which the seller promises to indemnify the retailer from lawsuits arising from a faulty product. It would be pointless to have this clause in code because it is not self-executing; rather, it remains to be read and implemented by a judge in the event of a lawsuit.

5.2.4. *Features of Blockchain*

Figure 5.2 depicts the characteristics of Blockchain technology.

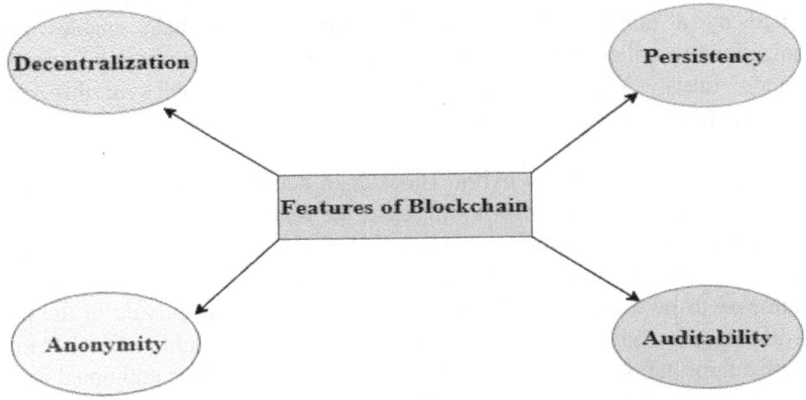

Figure 5.2. *Features of Blockchain. For a color version this figure, see www.iste.co.uk/choudhury/blockchain.zip*

Decentralization: in a typical centralized transaction system, each action must be verified by a single authorized organization. As a result, decentralization necessitates confidence, which is the most pressing problem, as well as raising durability, availability and failover, for which the decentralized P2P Blockchain framework may be a better fit (Bhushan et al. 2020). In the Blockchain network, a transaction may be made by any two peers (P2P) without the need for permission from a central agent. By using a variety of consensus procedures, Blockchain can help to alleviate confidence concerns. Furthermore, it will have lower processing costs (including production and operating costs) and eliminate bottlenecks in the core server's performance. Blockchain, on the contrary, has some tradeoffs in several ways. In PoW instances, such as Bitcoin and Ethereum, infrastructure and electricity expenses are in greater magnitude, but throughput is frequently orders of magnitude worse.

Persistency: Blockchain provides a platform for analyzing facts, enabling suppliers and consumers to establish that the data is credible and unaltered. If a Blockchain has 10 blocks, for instance, block number ten contains the hash of the previous matching block, and the content from the previous block is used to construct a new block. As a result, all of the blocks in the current chain are connected and joined. Furthermore, the transactions are linked to the prior one. A simple change to each transaction would now significantly modify the hash of the block. In addition, when a miner generates a block, it must be accepted by additional network participants. As a result, any information exploitation or fabrication will be detected by the system.

Anonymity: to connect with the Blockchain network, a dynamically generated address can be used. A user in a Blockchain network may have many addresses to ensure their identity. Because it is a decentralized structure, no one body monitors or records users' personal information. Because of its trustless setting, Blockchain offers some privacy.

Auditability: a software public register stores all events in a Blockchain network and verifies them with a digital timestamp. As a result, any networking node may be visited to examine and follow past records.

5.2.5. *Applications of Blockchain technology*

The Blockchain platform has a use in almost every sector. It is worth remembering that Bitcoin is not the same as Blockchain; rather, it is one of the more common uses of the technology (Memon et al. 2019). Some of the general applications of Blockchain technology are as follows.

Healthcare: healthcare can be transformed by distributed ledger technologies (McGhin et al. 2019). Blockchain will also help with drug tracking and clinical information safeguards. Drug piracy is a major problem in the healthcare companies. A fake drug is a drug or pharmacist item which is made and sold with the aim of deceiving its source, legitimacy or effectiveness. A counterfeit drug may have inadequate active chemicals, or nothing at all, and may be metabolized improperly in the body. According to the Health Research Funding Agency (Glass 2014), counterfeit pharmaceuticals account for 10–30% of all legal drugs in underdeveloped nations. Another big challenge for the healthcare sector is maintaining patient data confidentiality. Because all interactions are logged on a Blockchain, it has the potential to be a sustainable response to this issue. Unchangeable actions are added to the distributed ledger and electronically time-stamped, allowing for the tracking of an item's progression and making things tamper-proof by securing the information. Since each patient is different in terms of physical characteristics, a treatment plan for a common condition differs based on the circumstances. As a result, in order to get personalized care, it is important to give a link to the patient's symptoms. Medical data, on the contrary, is vulnerable and requires a stable sharing network. Blockchain technology, with its irreversible ledger, could provide a framework for the unification of patient history among multiple medical institutions, as well as data security measures. Blockchain is capable of providing a stable and open system for storing digital medical records, resulting in better patient care and lower treatment costs.

Energy Industry: one of the most extensively used Blockchain solutions in the energy business is microgrids. A microgrid is a locally integrated and regulated network of sources of electric power with the goal of increasing the efficiency and stability of energy generation and consumption. One of the most important benefits of microgrid technology is that it enables consumers and other electric power customers, like retailers, to not only access the electricity they need but also to sell and manufacture surplus energy to the grid. In microgrids, it is used to simplify, register and verify power sale and purchasing transactions. Similarly, at larger scales, Blockchain can be used to allow electricity sharing in smart grids. Blockchain can be used to facilitate safe and privacy-preserving usage control and electricity sharing without the requirements of the centralized person (Saxena et al. 2021).

Stock Market: interoperability, confidence and openness are all problems that fragmented business processes face. Blockchain technology may be able to address these issues. It will improve the stock exchange's efficiency by decentralizing and automating it. Blockchain will further cut costs by replacing intermediaries and speeding up contract settlements. Furthermore, the technology has the potential to be useful in contract clearance and settlement, as well as easing the tedious paperwork associated with trading and legal ownership transition and ensuring a safe post-trade mechanism.

Voting: Blockchain technology has several applications to solve issues that a traditional database may have. Voting is an example of such a dilemma. It was recently announced that a major voting machine maker in the United States had implemented remote control tools on some of their machines. When counting the totals, this program provided for the modification of votes. As a result of incidents like this, there is a loss of confidence in the election system of America: "Exclusive poll: The majority of people anticipate international meddling in the midterm elections". Because an elector's ledger is the same as the one used to count the votes, Blockchain can address this problem by creating a public ledger that ensures votes are recorded.

Insurance: Blockchain will be used to facilitate exchanges between clients, insurers and health insurers in the insurance business. Blockchain technology might be used by insurance companies to acquire and record contracts, file and evaluate complaints and pay premium operations. Smart contracts will simplify a variety of insurance plans, lowering management costs dramatically (Gatteschi et al. 2018).

Writing insurance claims, for example, comes with a heavy administrative expense. Owing to misunderstandings and misinterpretations of the terminology, the management of lawsuits may be a rather complicated procedure throughout several instances. By making insurance plans structured in more precise if-then partnerships, smart contracts will avoid these issues. These policies allow the implementation of terms to be automated by digital protocols. Insurance firms will lower the quality of their insurance premiums and become more attractive as a result of this cut, attracting more buyers.

5.3. Blockchain in healthcare

The Blockchain technology was created for its most well-known applications in economics and cryptocurrency, but its applications are increasing in different domains, including in biomedicine. Through stabilizing and protecting the data collection in which consumers can communicate through various forms of transactions, medication, biotechnology, telehealth, tele-monitoring, e-health, genetics and customized healthcare apps have all demonstrated promise for Blockchain technology. The sections that follow discuss specific domains of healthcare and medical care wherein Blockchain technology holds enormous potential.

Clinical research: in clinical trials, a variety of concerns such as data protection, integrity of data, sharing of data, patient enrollment and so on can occur. Blockchain, as the next internet generation, has the potential to solve these issues. With the assistance of Blockchain technologies, healthcare experts are trying to resolve these problems. Permission granted Ethereum is a Blockchain platform with smart contract features that is used in conjunction with systems for data computing centered in clinics. The major purpose of these studies is to overcome the patient enrollment conundrum.

Fraud detection: one of the most significant uses of Blockchain systems in the medical business is the control of pharmaceutical medication supply chains. Supply management is a key topic in many businesses, but it is especially vital in healthcare due to its increasing complexity. As a result, every disturbance in the supply chain of healthcare affects a patient's health. As a result of the many moving parts and individuals involved, supply chains are unstable and contain gaps for malicious assaults. Blockchains offer a safe and stable mechanism to eradicate this issue and, in some situations, avoid fraud from occurring.

Neuroscience: the amount of material and study devoted to Blockchain technology is continually growing, and neurology is unquestionably covered. The goal of advanced brain technology is to develop a modern system that removes mechanical disturbance in the setting and allows people to operate equipment and data, using mental instructions rather than physical ones. Such neural systems are capable of interpreting signals of activity related to brain and translating them into instructions for manipulating third party devices, along with predicting a person's current emotional state based on evidence from their brain activity. Around the same time, the device would "ensure protection and secrecy of personal information" so any abnormal behavior will be readily traceable.

Pharmaceutical research and industry: it is one of the world's fastest growing and a vital actor in healthcare delivery. At the production and R&D stages, Blockchain is employed for testing, monitoring and assuring the prospective manufacture of medications. Hyperledger, a research foundation, recently announced the start of a counterfeit medication initiative that will use Blockchain technology as the primary method for inspecting and combating the issue.

5.4. Electronic health records using Blockchain

Over the last decade, medical practitioners, clinics and medical products have also encouraged a growth in the digitalization of medical health records, since digitalization of this data provides for easier access and cooperation, as well as a basis for safer and faster making decisions. In the area of healthcare, the most common Blockchain solutions are currently in the field of EHR. As a result of life experiences that isolate them from one provider's data to another, patients' data is distributed among different organizations, and they lose simple access to previous data. A prototype known as "MedRec" (Azaria et al. 2016) makes use of unique Blockchain features to manage authentication, anonymity, honesty and data sharing. It is based on a decentralized system for the management of records that claims to provide patients with a detailed, permanent history as well as convenient access to their healthcare details from a variety of providers and treatment facilities. For MedRec, there is no reason to maintain patient records or wait for an adjustment time. It creates a Blockchain archive and notifies the client, who is entirely liable for the record's movement. The label ensures that a perfect copy of the record was obtained. Xia et al. (2017) developed MeDShare, a secure and reliable Blockchain architecture for the exchange of medical data between unknown individuals.

EHRs often include highly sensitive and critical patient data that is exchanged on a regular basis by doctors, radiologists, hospital employees, chemists and scientists in order to give correct diagnosis and treatment. The collection and distribution of this very personal patient information to various entities can endanger the patient's care, posing major threats to the patient's health and the capacity to maintain an up-to-date patient record. Consequently, maintaining an up-to-date patient's history has become vital to ensure effective care. To overcome these challenges, a

Blockchain-based network for keeping, maintaining and transferring electronic medical information for cancer patients should be developed. To view, handle and archive secure patient data, they used permissioned Blockchain technology. These proposed solutions will be used to incorporate Blockchain technologies in healthcare practices for maintaining the safety and confidentiality of information of patient and background. Perhaps the explanation for the rapid adoption of Blockchain technologies in medicine around the world is a clear promise to patients that using this technology can make their medical data permanent and unaltered. Any access or modification initiative may be easily branded and identified through the Blockchain. This is valuable not only for medical integrity, but it also flags some fraudulent activities, such as wholesale bribery or record adulteration. Furthermore, posting and reviewing authorized medicinal service records would be much easier. When a patient visits, the rest of the patient's suppliers are likely to notice it right away. Pharmaceutical errors, hypersensitivities and pharmaceutical solutions may be seamlessly related across all Blockchain records using suitable patient-caring algorithms, removing the need for time-consuming prescriptions agreement forms. As a result, the application of Blockchain technology would improve treatment accessibility, medical record management, quick clinical proof verification, greater monitoring and more effective healthcare management.

Al-Karaki et al. (2019) have presented a DASS-CARE that is a Blockchain-based system that enables open connectivity to health centers, particularly medical information, that is scalable and secure. The proposed system would significantly simplify the process of real-time access and notifications without jeopardizing patient data protection, integrity or confidentiality.

Vora et al. (2019) developed a system based on Blockchain for EHR storage and maintenance that is both effective and safe. The suggested system also enables customers, providers and other organizations to connect to medical data in a secure and convenient manner while maintaining patient confidentiality.

Dagher et al. (2018) developed a system based on Blockchain for patients, insurers and third parties to offer secure, accessible and dependable connectivity to health data while protecting patients' personal information.

5.5. Quantitative analysis

Quantitative analysis is concerned with describing and comprehending things statistically and quantitatively. The purpose of quantitative analysis is to comprehend the data collected for the phenomenon via the use of numerical variables and analytics. Quantitative analysis includes statistical and analytical approaches of analysis.

We examined the Scopus database for research published up until November 1, 2021. Studies on Blockchain-based electronic health records (EHRs) have been published not just in medical publications, but also in journals from other fields such as IT, law, engineering, economics and business administration. As a result, given its comprehensive coverage of journals in both the scientific and social sciences, we chose the Scopus database as the source of papers for this study.

We employed four processes to conduct a comprehensive quantitative review: discovering possible research, removing unnecessary research, verifying important studies and evaluating selected articles.

In the first phase of selecting suitable research, we conducted a preliminary search for papers that had a term like "electronic health record" in their titles, abstracts or keywords. This phase yielded a total of 70,616 prospective investigations. In a separate search, we limited these studies to those that had key phrases like "Blockchain electronic health records" in their titles, abstracts or keywords. This resulted in a total of 500 prospective research.

In the second phase, a filter is applied to remove the articles in press which yields the 484 documents out of 500 documents. The Scopus database also shows the articles in press which means that the articles are not published yet online but are in the production stage.

In the third phase of verifying the significance of the 484 available studies, we probed their document types, titles, abstracts and keywords, and filtered out 464 studies that satisfied the set of criteria of our search with the publication in English language alone. This stage approved 464 articles in total.

In the fourth phase of analyzing the 464 articles, we looked at how they were distributed by publication year, language, location of origination, journal and yearly average number of citations. The nations of origin of the publications were studied by identifying the countries of the organization to which the authors belonged. If an article had two writers working for organizations in two distinct nations, the country of origin was determined to be two countries. The top 10 articles were determined using the yearly average number of citations of the 464 articles. When corrected for the effects of time after publication, the yearly average number of citations can more precisely indicate the amount of influence of each item on other research than the overall number of citations. A 2016 article, for instance, is more likely to be mentioned than one produced in 2019. As a result, we ranked the 464 publications using the yearly average number of citations.

5.5.1. *Results*

The quantity of articles has skyrocketed since 2016. Out of all these articles, only two were published in 2016. From 2017, the number of articles is continuously increasing in the domain of Blockchain-based EHRs. Figure 5.3 shows the rise in the number of articles from 2016 to 2021 till date.

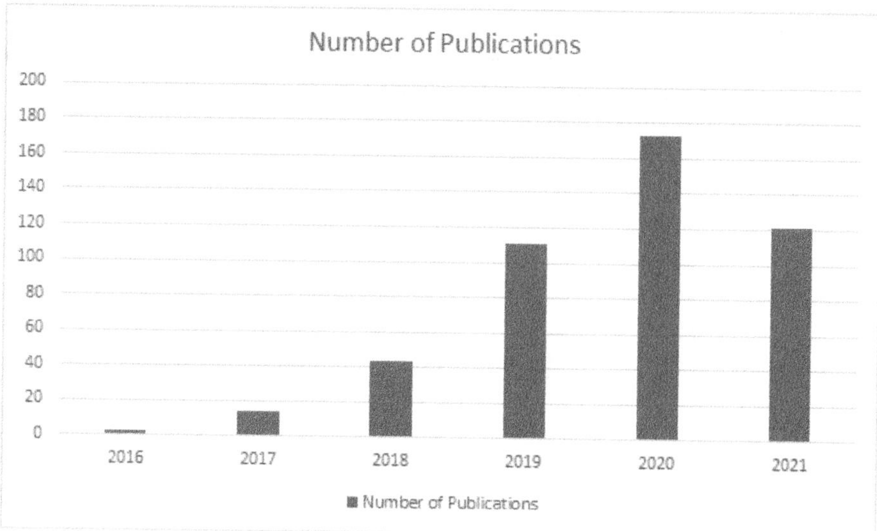

Figure 5.3. *Number of publications*

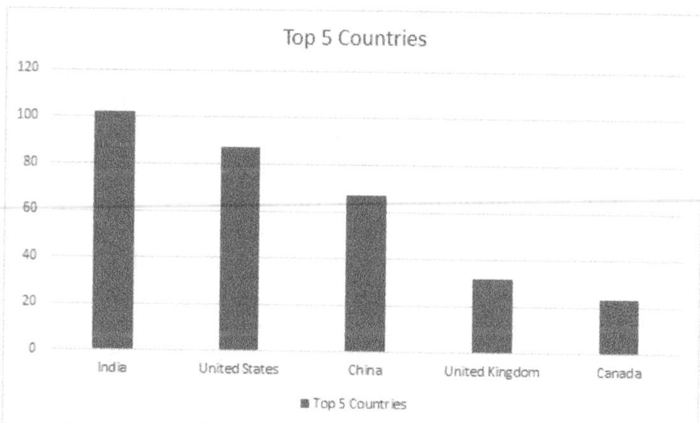

Figure 5.4. *Top 5 countries in terms of publications*

India, the United States, China, the United Kingdom and Canada are the top 5 countries in terms of the number of articles published. India has the maximum number of articles, that is 102, which constitutes around 21.9% of the selected articles for review. Figure 5.4 shows the top 5 countries.

IEEE Access, Journal of Medical Internet Research, Journal of Medical Systems, Advances in Intelligent Systems and Computing and Lecture Notes in Computer Science Including Subseries Lecture Notes in Artificial Intelligence and Lecture Notes in Bioinformatics are the top 5 sources in terms of number of publications. IEEE Access has the maximum number of documents that is 26. Figure 5.5 shows the top 5 sources.

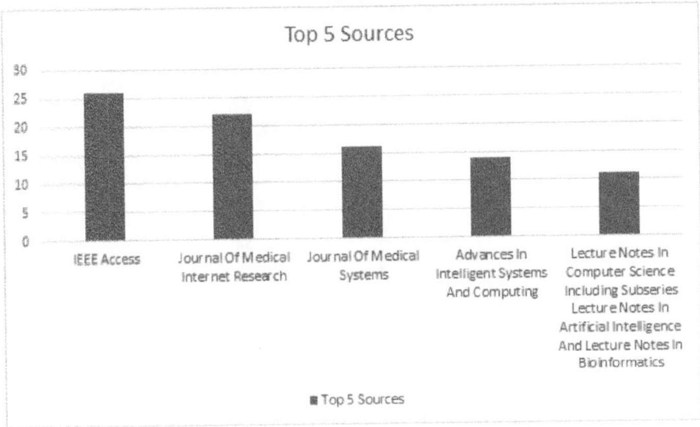

Figure 5.5. *Top 5 sources in terms of number of publications*

The goal of quantitative research is to learn about and comprehend the social world. Social scientists, particularly communication academicians, employ quantitative analysis to analyze occurrences or occurrings which effect humans. The quantitative analysis described above enables researchers to do simple or complex investigations, such as showing data links, calculating averages or percentages, or using inferential statistics to draw broad generalizations about a large population. This research will be useful to academicians and practitioners interested in Blockchain technology for maintaining EHRs and those who are looking for collaboration opportunities with other academicians and research institutions by carefully collecting, categorizing and evaluating research publications related to Blockchain-based EHR.

5.6. Proposed framework for the EHRs using Blockchain

This segment introduces the proposed solution for EHR sharing, which is built on the Blockchain network. For block transactions in the network, various methods and configurations are used. This section describes the Blockchain-based EHR system architecture. The proposed scheme has six members. The entities involved are: patients, doctors, administrative staff, insurance company, lab technicians and pharmacies.

– Administrative staff: the administrative staff is responsible for registering the users into the Blockchain. They register the users on the Blockchain and provide permissions to the users.

– Doctor: the doctor is responsible for adding the medical details of the patient to the Blockchain. The doctor is also authorized to view the details of the patient.

– Patient: the patient is responsible to add the previous medical details. The patient is also authorized to insert the new medical record.

– Lab technician: the lab technician is responsible to add the test reports of the patient. They cannot access the patient's medical details.

– Pharmacy: the pharmacy owner is responsible for delivering the required medicines to the patient. He is able to view the prescription uploaded by the doctor. The pharmacy owner cannot access the medical details of the patient.

– Insurance company: the insurance company is responsible for settling the hospital bills of the patient. The insurance company can only view the hospital bills of the patient uploaded by the administrative staff of the hospital.

5.6.1. *System workflow*

Figure 5.6 shows the workings of the proposed model.

Firstly, the administrative staff registers the patient on the Blockchain by the registration smart contract. Once the patient is registered, the administrative staff registers the particular doctor and grants permission via the smart contract. After the registration process is completed, the doctor provides the treatment to the patient and continuously updates the records on the Blockchain network. The doctor is not able to delete the particular record on the Blockchain. Once the initial medication is done, the doctor recommends lab tests to the patient. The patient conveys the lab information to the administrative staff so that only an authorized lab technician is able to update the record on the Blockchain. Once the test is done, the authorized lab technician is able to upload the reports that can be accessed by the authorized doctor. Once the treatment is done, the doctor will upload the prescription on the

Blockchain network. The patient conveys the pharmacy owner details to the administrative staff so that only authorized persons get the prescription details. The healthcare store proprietor obtains the medication history and brings the medications to the healthcare center. Once all the treatment is done, the administrative staff uploads the bill on the Blockchain network and it is not modifiable by the patient. The patient conveys all the details about the insurance to the administrative staff so that the legitimate insurance company can view the bills of the patient and process the claim. The insurance company is not authorized to view the medical details of the patient. In this way, the claim process will be settled without any fraud.

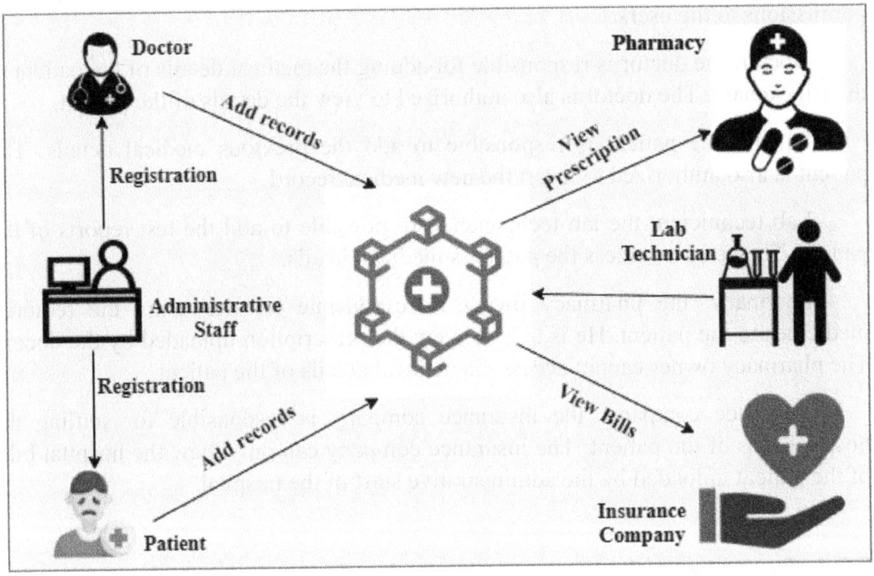

Figure 5.6. *Proposed model. For a color version this figure, see www.iste.co.uk/choudhury/blockchain.zip*

5.7. Issues in Blockchain-based EHRs

The EHR Blockchain literature has described interoperability, anonymity and authorization (access control) as major issues and challenges.

Interoperability issues between insurer and healthcare networks contribute to the difficulty of effectively exchanging data (Monrat et al. 2019). Health reports are scattered rather than coherent due to less organized management of data and sharing. Many studies have raised questions about data interoperability and fragmentation.

Since EHR data, including photographs, can be quite vast in size, scalability is a major challenge when transmitting EHR data through Blockchain. Because of a Blockchain network's distributed replicated existence, saving and duplicating EHR data on the network for redistribution is difficult due to the massive data volume.

The current EHRs have very few patient management permissions, and patients are usually unable to freely exchange their data with researchers or providers. Despite all of medicine's advancements, multiple EHR mechanisms are unable to interact efficiently.

5.8. Case studies

5.8.1. *MedRec*

MedRec is a framework that promotes patient agency by providing direct and open access to medical experience, therefore bridging a societal need with a technological enabler. To extend the banking model, financial systems may have a variety of currency storage facilities, such as one for each network of providers. The issue is that medical files are not interchangeable; each one has a person's signature. There is no such thing as a like-for-like exchange of money. Although competition and variety may lower market pricing, they typically risk creating a cascade of unsuitable or inaccessible exchange and control obstacles. To circumvent arbitrary middlemen, developers have developed a distributed access and validation approach that leverages the Blockchain.

Members of a proprietary, P2P network share data control and viewership permits, which are reflected in the block content in MedRec. Smart contracts, which are made possible by Blockchain technology, assist the users in automating and monitoring certain state transitions. The developers use smart contracts on the Ethereum Blockchain to monitor the relationship of provider and patient, which link a medical record to accessing privileges and information retrieval directions for implementation on the Blockchain. Patients can consent to the sharing of information across providers. In all situations, the individual collecting new data receives an automatic update and has the opportunity to examine the suggested input before accepting or rejecting it. This allows users to stay up to date on the progress of their papers. MedRec prioritizes accessibility by offering a contract that gathers changes any of a recipient's client interactions, as well as a central source of contact for looking for health record updates. Figure 5.7 shows the workings of the MedRec system.

MedRec's block information represents ownership rights and viewing privileges maintained by users of a private, P2P system. Scientists use Ethereum smart contracts to register patient interactions by associating a health file with reading rights and data retrieval commands (essentially data pointers) for implementation on other systems. To ensure data integrity, the investigators upload a cryptographic hash of the item to the Blockchain to avoid manipulation. Consumers can authorize the sharing of records among doctors, and suppliers can create a new record linked to a particular client. The researchers validate identity using public key cryptography and a DNS-like solution to link a genuine and widely accepted kind of ID to the individual's Ethereum address.

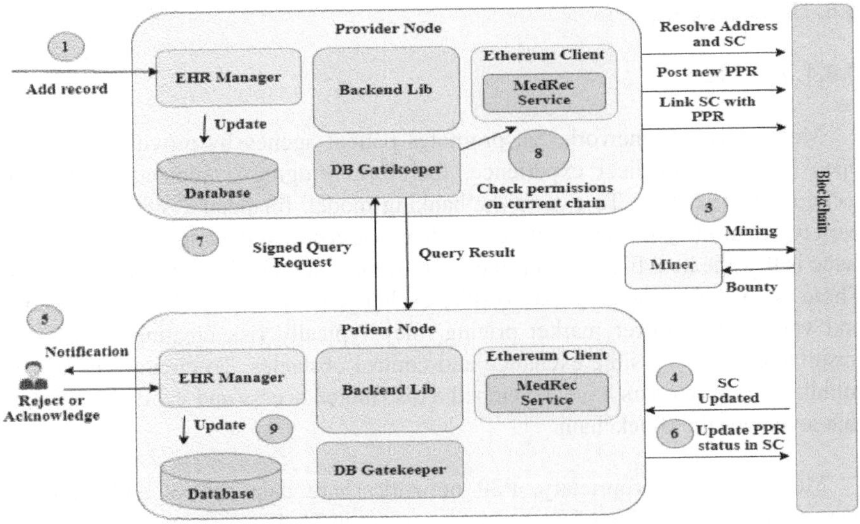

Figure 5.7. *Working of MedRec (Xia et al. 2017). For a color version this figure, see www.iste.co.uk/choudhury/blockchain.zip*

5.8.2. *AI-based solution for EHRs*

An Artificial Intelligence (AI)-enabled and Blockchain-driven EHR management platform has immense potential to support trustworthy, secure and resilient EHR storage services. This sort of EHR system would also make it simpler for academics, physicians and officials to obtain data for research, perform analysis and make sound decisions.

Mistry et al. (2021) presented MedBlock, an AI-enabled and Blockchain-powered secure EHR solution for safeguarding the privacy of Covid-19 positive patients. It involves a number of organizations, including physicians, staff workers, public officials, hospitals and consumers. Data transfer in the MedBlock is allowed by using the Ethereum network only if it fits the parameters of the smart contract. MedBlock also ensures that EHRs are not manipulated with or used for malicious reasons. Since information transmission of Covid-19 patients was crucial in the pandemic, the proposed system used a 6G network channel of communication, which reduced information transmission latency (10–100 sec) and reliability (99.99999%). The layers of MedBlock are as follows: (i) data collection and aggregation, (ii) AI, (iii) Blockchain and (iv) accessibility. The data collected and aggregated by the preceding layer is sent into the AI layer. The AI makes decisions based on the data provided. The Artificial Neural Network (ANN) receives the patient's Covid-19 laboratory and CT-Scan results. It functions as a binary classifier based on the input parameters. The ANN model is used to determine whether the patient is positive or negative for Covid-19. The EHR, which can be either positive or negative, is an input to the layer that follows. Algorithm 5.1 depicts the step-by-step approach for AI-based Covid-19 patient categorization.

Input: α is the number of data entries in the dataset Π with maximum δ entries. Π_X and Πy are the X_{train}(input) and Y_{train}(required – output), that are employed for the aim of training.

Output: Training for Classifiers

procedure CLASSIFIERTRAINING(X_{train}, Y_{train})

while (True) do

applyPCA(α, ncomponents = optimalnumber)

Choose the best number for the main components.

if (isNull(Π)) then

Return ("Enter the training data.");

else if ($\alpha > \delta$) then

EndTraining();

ModelTestonTestData();

else

$\alpha = \alpha + 1$;

```
trainingANNonTrainingData(Xtrain, ytrain);
ρ = Πrecord            //Here the ρ is the record
ObtainNextData(Π, ρ);
Continue;
end if
end If
end while
end procedure
```

Algorithm 5.1. *Training procedure based on AI (Mistry et al. 2021):*

5.8.3. *Improving medical record keeping with Blockchain*

phrOS (phrOS – Healthcare Blockchain Operating System) was recently launched by Taipei Medical University Hospital and Digital Treasury Corporation (DTCO) (see DTCO n.d.). It attempts to promote openness among medical organizations by storing all of a patient's medical records on a Blockchain. It contains photos as well as numerous pieces of information on a patient's condition. A smartphone app allows clinicians and patients to view the information. It also improves the security of medical data by using Decentralized Ledger Technology (DLT). The open framework allows for autonomous and secure solutions, making smart health a reality. It generates an anonymized digital identity for patients to aid in patient verification and identification, as well as patient data recording and querying, covering in treatment and medication planning. Smart contracts can be used in clinical trials for protocol changes, trial enrollment delays and so on. Patient-authorized claims, including timestamps and medical records, as well as all authorized files, have digital signatures that can be evaluated at any time without the need for third-party services to resolve conflicts.

5.9. Conclusion

The usage of Blockchain in application areas is critical in today's healthcare business. It might lead to autonomous data collection and authentication procedures, as well as trustworthy and integrated information from several sources that is long-lasting, tamper-resistant and safe, with a lower risk of theft. In this chapter, the framework for EHR based on Blockchain is proposed. The primary purpose is to apply Blockchain technology to EHRs by addressing its key properties in order to provide tamper-proof, distributed, irrevocable, transparent, reliable, and open to scrutiny remote medical care. Furthermore, the chapter discussed the potential benefits of Blockchain technology in medical systems. It also includes a discussion of the current Blockchain-based electronic health records that doctors use to store health data. The chapter finishes with a list of challenges that must be solved in order to improve the electronic health record system through the use of upcoming Blockchain-based networks.

5.10. References

Aggarwal, S., Chaudhary, R., Aujla, G.S., Kumar, N., Choo, K.K.R., Zomaya, A.Y. (2019). Blockchain for smart communities: Applications, challenges and opportunities. *Journal of Network and Computer Applications*, 144, 13–48. DOI: 10.1016/J.JNCA.2019.06.018.

Al-Karaki, J.N., Gawanmeh, A., Ayache, M., Mashaleh, A. (2019). DASS-CARE: A decentralized, accessible, scalable, and secure healthcare framework using blockchain. *2019 15th International Wireless Communications and Mobile Computing Conference*, IWCMC 2019 330–335. DOI: 10.1109/IWCMC.2019.8766714.

Andreev, R.A., Andreeva, P.A., Krotov, L.N., Krotova, E.L. (2018). Review of Blockchain technology: Types of Blockchain and their application. *Intellektual'nye sistemy v proizvodstve*, 16, 11. DOI: 10.22213/2410-9304-2018-1-11-14.

Azaria, A., Ekblaw, A., Vieira, T., Lippman, A. (2016). MedRec: Using Blockchain for medical data access and permission management. *Proceedings – 2016 2nd International Conference on Open and Big Data*, OBD 2016 25–30. DOI: 10.1109/OBD.2016.11.

Bhushan, B., Khamparia, A., Sagayam, K.M., Sharma, S.K., Ahad, M.A., Debnath, N.C. (2020). Blockchain for smart cities: A review of architectures, integration trends and future research directions. *Sustainable Cities and Society*, 61, 102360. DOI: 10.1016/J.SCS.2020.102360.

Dagher, G.G., Mohler, J., Milojkovic, M., Marella, P.B. (2018). Ancile: Privacy-preserving framework for access control and interoperability of electronic health records using blockchain technology. *Sustainable Cities and Society*, 39, 283–297. DOI: 10.1016/J.SCS.2018.02.014.

DTCO (n.d.) phrOS – Healthcare Blockchain operating system [Online]. Available at: https://phros.io/ [Accessed 12 July 22].

Gatteschi, V., Lamberti, F., Demartini, C., Pranteda, C., Santamaría, V. (2018). Blockchain and smart contracts for insurance: Is the technology mature enough? *Future Internet*, 10(2), 20. DOI: 10.3390/FI10020020.

Glass, B.D. (2014). Counterfeit drugs and medical devices in developing countries. *Research and Reports in Tropical Medicine*, 5, 11. DOI: 10.2147/RRTM.S39354.

Jani, S. (2020). Smart contracts: Building blocks for digital transformation. DOI: 10.13140/RG.2.2.33316.83847.

Katal, A., Sethi, V., Lamba, S. (2021a). Blockchain consensus algorithms: Study and challenges. *EAI/Springer Innovations in Communication and Computing*, 45–64. DOI: 10.1007/978-3-030-65691-1_4/COVER/.

Katal, A., Singh, J., Kundnani, Y. (2021b). Mitigating the effects of fake news using blockchain and machine learning. *2021 2nd International Conference for Emerging Technology*, INCET 2021. DOI: 10.1109/INCET51464.2021.9456205.

McGhin, T., Choo, K.K.R., Liu, C.Z., He, D. (2019). Blockchain in healthcare applications: Research challenges and opportunities. *Journal of Network and Computer Applications*, 135, 62–75. DOI: 10.1016/J.JNCA.2019.02.027.

Memon, M., Hussain, S.S., Bajwa, U.A., Ikhlas, A. (2019). Blockchain beyond Bitcoin: Blockchain technology challenges and real-world applications. *Proceedings – 2018 International Conference on Computing, Electronics and Communications Engineering, iCCECE 2018*, 29–34. DOI: 10.1109/ICCECOME.2018.8658518.

Mistry, C., Thakker, U., Gupta, R., Obaidat, M.S., Tanwar, S., Kumar, N., Rodrigues, J.J.P.C. (2021). MedBlock: An AI-enabled and Blockchain-driven medical healthcare system for Covid-19. *IEEE International Conference on Communications*. DOI: 10.1109/ICC42927.2021.9500397.

Monrat, A.A., Schelén, O., Andersson, K. (2019). A survey of Blockchain from the perspectives of applications, challenges, and opportunities. *IEEE Access*, 7, 117134–117151. DOI: 10.1109/ACCESS.2019.2936094.

Saxena, S., Bhushan, B., Ahad, M.A. (2021). Blockchain based solutions to secure IoT: Background, integration trends and a way forward. *Journal of Network and Computer Applications*, 181, 103050. DOI: 10.1016/J.JNCA.2021.103050.

Vora, J., Nayyar, A., Tanwar, S., Tyagi, S., Kumar, N., Obaidat, M.S., Rodrigues, J.J.P.C. (2019). BHEEM: A Blockchain-based framework for securing electronic health records. *2018 IEEE Globecom Workshops, GC Wkshps 2018 – Proceedings*. DOI: 10.1109/GLOCOMW.2018.8644088.

Xia, Q., Sifah, E.B., Asamoah, K.O., Gao, J., Du, X., Guizani, M. (2017). MeDShare: Trust-less medical data sharing among cloud service providers via Blockchain. *IEEE Access*, 5, 14757–14767. DOI: 10.1109/ACCESS.2017.2730843.

Zhang, Y., Deng, R.H., Liu, X., Zheng, D. (2018). Blockchain based efficient and robust fair payment for outsourcing services in cloud computing. *Information Sciences*, 462, 262–277. DOI: 10.1016/J.INS.2018.06.018.

6

An Optimistic Approach to Share Private Health Records Using Blockchain Technology

These days, the amount of digital health data generated is increasing. Legacy systems with confidentiality and security problems are used to store and share them. Insurance data, banking information and Electronic Health Records (EHRs) are all examples of sensitive data or documents that must be exchanged digitally. Because EHRs include vital information and are frequently exchanged among several parties, including hospitals, patients and government bodies, they are both critical and sensitive. Private clinics or pharmacies maintain this information to be accurate, up to date, secret and made accessible to authorized users. In many circumstances, the transaction takes place between anonymous and unreliable people. As a result, implementing the data exchange using a fair non-repudiation protocol is considerably critical. Blockchain is no longer exclusively associated with cryptocurrencies such as Bitcoin. Blockchain is now widely used in applications that require immutable and traceable data, as well as a cryptographic and distributed ledger and is most often used in secure transactions. In a distributed ledger, records are maintained in a linked sequence of blocks, known as a Blockchain. The proposed system connects with the methods such as on-chain and off-chain communication patterns to allow patients and healthcare professionals to share personal health records. A scheme that emphasizes the importance of maintaining a true fair-exchange policy while transferring medical records without the involvement of a trusted third party is proposed. This distributed technology has a lot of potential in new applications over dissimilar fields such as healthcare and stakeholders.

6.1. Introduction

Blockchain, according to the current study, has the potential to dislocate trusted business models that are mostly used in present day healthcare systems that perform

For a color version of all figures in this chapter, see www.iste.co.uk/choudhury/blockchain.zip.
Chapter written by P. PRAVEEN, Mohammed Ali SHAIK, B. RAMA and V. ANITHA.

information sharing (Ethereum n.d.; Esposito et al. 2018). Given the amount of transactions (sharing of information), including various healthcare objects and the costs that incur in Hospital Maintenance Systems (HIE), using Blockchain technologies that democratically sustain in various public ledgers are recorded with various novel and inspiring prospects in the healthcare industry. The Blockchain technology has the ability to build an electronic environment in which people perform various business transactions (information sharing) through a disseminated community instead of a central authority. This could have a big impact on how transparent the system is and the functions of each institution (Dias et al. 2018; Ravi Kumar et al. 2019). By improving exchange of information along with coordination with various healthcare groups, Blockchain can also help individuals become more self-sufficient in sharing their medical records with clinicians. Based on the scale, most of the mainstream HIE servers are coordinated by huge enterprises or institutions of healthcare. Centralized administration may introduce privacy and security issues due to the abuse of authority, such as ancillary use of medical records and their unapproved access, or even hacker attacks. Blockchain technology, on the contrary, may support a range of characteristics such as decentralization.

Most of the studies looking at the consequences of Blockchain-based distributed ledger technology for performing healthcare practices have generated a lot of interest (Dai et al. 2020; Feng et al. 2020). However, little quantitative study has been done on HIE's use of Blockchain technology. Patients' opinions for enabling the deployment of Blockchain-based HIE networks are unknown and it is unclear whether patients (HIE stakeholders) will support its use. As a result, most of the research needed to evaluate the principal implementation of Blockchain technology over the healthcare industry is from the patient's point of view. This chapters findings can help healthcare organizations or communities and politicians clearly understand the use of Blockchain technology in recognizing various incorporated benefits and risks in healthcare practices (Blum et al. 1988; Crameri et al. 2020).

6.2. Related work

In Blockchain-based EHR systems, most of the steps involved in improvising the privacy protection of complex health records as privacy preserving methods can be divided into cryptographic and non-cryptographic categories, with encryption or anonymization and access control mechanisms as examples (Praveen and Jayanth Babu 2019).

Encryption schemes, for instance, Public Key Encryption (PKE), Symmetric Key Encryption (SKE), secure Multi Party Computation (MPC) and others are rather widespread. In the proposed system, a Blockchain based in a healthcare network comprises a public key encryption technique, such as Elliptic Curve Cryptography (ECC). This is used to perform the encryption of private data over a secure channel, which corresponds to the data generated from various sensors that will be uploaded in a Blockchain network by means of a pair of exclusive private and public keys, in order to ensure the privacy and security of biometric data (Daemen and Rijmen 2002; Dai et al. 2020).

Al Omar et al. (2017) advocated that data should be encrypted using a symmetric key technique with a threshold encryption scheme before being uploaded to cloud services. The process of Shamir's Secret Sharing (SSS) divides the symmetric key into many shares that are further distributed to distinct key keepers. The process of decrypting the encrypted text can be performed when the data requestor accepts adequate key segments. Data leaking may not arise when certain key keepers negotiate the (minimal threshold) value. Smart phone is a Healthcare Data Gateway (HDG) that is built on Blockchain, and uses MPC technology by enabling the system that calculates the data that is encrypted directly by performing over the private Blockchain cloud, to attain the concluding results instead of illuminating original data (Azaria et al. 2016; Ahsan et al. 2020).

Changing encryption keys is a common practice in healthcare systems and is a common method to avoid malicious, statistical attacks. But it incurs enhanced storing and managing costs with a large number of historical keys, which should be stored properly in sequence to perform decryption of some historical data in near future. This process leads to an increase in storage costs, specifically because of partial computational means and storage procedures to solve problems such as: web developed trivial backup and recovery key management systems that are implemented as a body of sensor networks (BSNs) to protect the privacy of the sensor data from a person by reducing secret key storage expenses. Without storing any encryption keys, fuzzy vault technology is used to generate, backup and recover keys, with BSNs performing the key recovery of the sensor data that is encrypted using symmetric encryption technology (AES or 3DES) (Blum et al. 1988; Rama et al. 2017). Hence, the attacker will have a hard time decrypting it without a symmetric key.

6.2.1. *Process of storing larger healthcare data*

By using EHR systems, medical records and other data can be easily uploaded based on the block size, which is fixed and limited as the data in Blockchain network is raised while performing computational overheads, to protect the storage subject from privacy breaches.

Over a period of time, the maximum frequency of cloud storage, which is continuously encrypted dynamic data attained from distinct available devices that emit transactions to Blockchain over the health data, can be obtained for machine learning data. The same can be further decrypted when the buyer allows us to share keys, as the architecture is capable of elevating the restriction of Blockchain by allowing precise rollbacks with enhanced false alarm rates. The offline databases were also used as a cache for medical data, with a database gatekeeper who was given permission if requested as they can return the query results (Benchoufi and Ravaud 2017).

It is a system in which the basic materials safeguard the security and privacy of data that is verified and signed by EHR, using healthcare that provides attribute-based signatures by trusting the third-party database (Rama et al. 2017; Praveen and Jayanth Babu 2019).

6.3. Blockchain-based EHR system

Further important aims are defined in the deployment of a secure Blockchain created on EHR schemes, with the requirements of a novel version for protected EHR systems and various features of the Blockchain stated earlier:

– *Confidentiality*: individual data will be used in a private manner and only authorized persons will have access to the required information.

– *Security (CIA)*: in terms of confidentiality, integrity and availability:

1) *Confidentiality*: data can only be accessed by authorized individuals.

2) *Integrity*: when the data is in transit it must be accurate and must not be tampered with by the unauthorized party.

3) *Availability*: the information and resources that are to be accessed by lawful users cannot be improperly denied.

– *Auditability*: a crucial aspect of security. For example, audit logs primarily contain statistical evidence of who has access to the EHR (PHR) for the purpose and time stamping performed by any process throughout the life-cycle.

– *Accountability*: a person or an organization will be assessed and held accountable for their actions.

– *Authenticity*: the capacity to verify requestor identities before granting entry to complex data.

– *Anonymity*: for privacy, entities take no apparent identity as absolute anonymity is difficult to achieve. Pseudo anonymity is more widespread, with the use of actual identities. Prevailing Blockchain grounded research in the field of healthcare involves the following essential features in order to meet the above goals.

– *Data archiving*: the Blockchain is a considerably reliable ledger database, which is used to accumulate a diversity of private healthcare information by securing the storage and guaranteeing data privacy.

– *Collaboration on data*: in most of the prevailing healthcare systems, almost all of the package contributors are typically the principal data custodians. The aspect of self-sovereignty provides ownership of healthcare data to every user who wants to share personal data is widespread today, hence it is very important to attain safe data sharing across various enterprises and domains.

– *Audit of data when conflicts emerge*: the audit logs can be used as documentation to hold requestors who are accountable for their interactions with EHRs. A wide range of systems tend to use Blockchain and smart contracts that keep track by recording all of the transactions with auditability of the Blockchain ledger that is accessible at any time.

– *Manage your identity*: in the system, the legitimacy of each user identity has to be ensured to protect system security and avoid malicious attacks, which makes it possible for legitimate users to make further appropriate requests.

We will look at existing methods for data storage, data sharing, data auditing and identity management in the rest of this section.

However, having complete reliance on third parties to keep the subtle information is risky. For the moment, it may be incompatible with the principle of decentralization, and to speed up the implementation of distributed storage systems like IPFS in the real world, more research is required. The next stage is to perform the design of the Blockchain storage architecture with elevated storage capability.

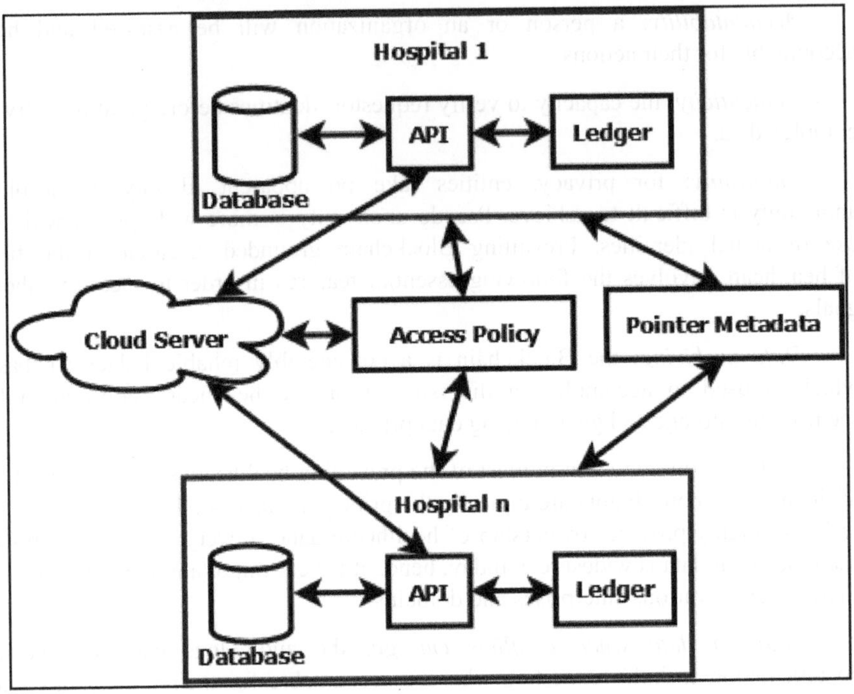

Figure 6.1. *Architecture diagram*

6.3.1. *Sharing of data*

Hospitals, clinics, laboratories and other healthcare facilities rely on a range of data sources maintained in diverse systems, as the healthcare data has to be preserved then recovered and altered through various healthcare contributors for medical objectives that include medical data that interchange. The adapted technique is problematic due to the diverse data architecture between different institutions. It is considerably critical to ensure data interoperability among different entities before sharing the data.

6.3.2. *Interoperability*

In the present-day era, the level of an EHR is assumed and implemented by most of the distinct contributors when they recite each of the additional data. This is known as interoperability, whose process can be effectively employed by standardizing and improvising the healthcare superiority, which is further classified into three groupings:

– Syntactic interoperability: the appropriate process that permits one EHR format system to associate with additional system.

– Semantic interoperability: the process of data sharing with appropriate data that has to be translated in between distinct systems at the data field level.

– Interoperability across domains: when we consider distinct organizations that cooperate to confirm protected and appropriate data communication as the effective data that is being used between various organizations and individuals.

6.3.3. *A distributed network*

The architecture being implemented in Blockchain is a peer-to-peer (P2P) architecture that consists of distinct nodes made up of various network participants, where each of the associates in the network stores a duplicate copy of the Blockchain and provides for cooperative procedures to further validate and certify all of the digital transactions in the network.

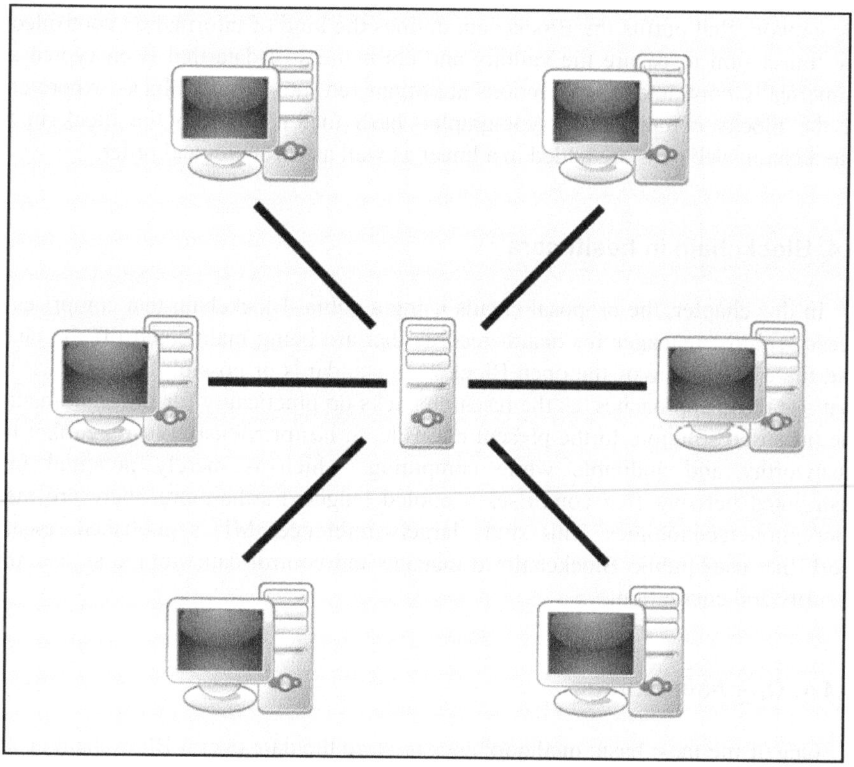

Figure 6.2. *Blockchain P-to-P architecture*

6.3.4. *Shared ledger*

Various members in the distributed network will tend to record all of the digital transactions in a shared ledger by implementing various algorithms for evaluating and verifying the proposed transactions. In the process for every novel, transaction is supplementary over the collective ledger when the majority of the network participants accept the transaction which is valid. Modifications in the collective ledger are replicated over all the duplicates of Blockchain within an acceptable amount of time in most of the situations that occur. By definition, every transaction is immutable and combined with the ledger, which cannot be further modified or withdrawn, as every member of the network has a widespread and clear model of the Blockchain and no specific person has the ability to damage or modify the data in this technology.

6.3.5. *Digital transactions*

In a Blockchain, any kind of information or digital quality can be recorded, and the network that outfits the Blockchain defines the kind of information controlled in the transaction to ensure the validity and correctness of data that is encrypted and numerically contracted. Transactions are organized into distinct blocks, where each of the blocks comprises a cryptographic hash that is prior to the block in the Blockchain, as blocks are added in a linear as well as chronological order.

6.4. Blockchain in healthcare

In this chapter, the proposal entails using a public Blockchain that comprises an access control manager for health records that are being maintained off the chain, and there exist none of the open Blockchain standards or possible implementations that use these approaches, as the research backs up practicality for the attainment of the proposed solution. In the present era, Bitcoin has previously illustrated that it is trustworthy and auditable while computing, which is merely potential in a distributed network that comprises a pooled ledger. Furthermore, there are many encryption technologies. This study largely references MIT's published research work that uses public Blockchain to manage and control data storage access, then security and encryption.

6.4.1. *On-chain storage*

One of the most basic methodologies to store the data over a Blockchain is very simply to chain the data itself as binary data, which can be kept as a fragment of a transaction that is subsequently disseminated for the community with the possible and available transactions. This process elevates the dilemma about the maximum amount of data that can be stored in one Blockchain over the transactions. Bitcoin is considerably the most valued cryptocurrency with a fixed block size Blockchain. The concept of Bitcoin with a semi-fixed block size comprised of 1 megabyte itself received a lot of attention. Theoretically, the definite size of the block, which can be in between 1 megabyte and somewhat larger, will be semi-fixed and not be hard-fixed. In a single block size, there will be an inadequate number of transactions to be deposited in a specific block with a single source of contention, and when end-users are forced to pay large transaction fees may result in a huge impact, due to the present popularity of Bitcoin pairing.

6.4.2. *Off-chain storage*

On-chain storage is considerably neither economically nor precisely feasible as most of the Blockchain benefits can be used for off-chain storage solutions. The hash of a small bit of data, for example, can be placed in the chain. Because a hash is very modest in size, the cost of storage will be low as well. The task then becomes establishing a link between the chain's hash and the physical storage place. Smart contracts and distributed hash tables (DHT) are comprised of dual solutions that are examined in this regard. In this instance, the data is also lost, and there is no way to restore it. Hash tables and distributed hash tables have a few ways to get around the drawbacks of using clever agreements for humble peer-to-peer storage and use numerous models of files in a storage network, so that even if the unique storage site becomes unreachable, the data is available everywhere. This eliminates the place as a unique point of disappointment for the data as the major concern of scattered hash tables is a resultant of (DHT).

6.4.3. *Trust issues in the context of health information exchange (HIE)*

The aspect of trust is critical in situations when consumers and sellers are separated based on Internet-based environments (Carvalho et al. 2016). Most of the HIE networks tend to share patient's health information electronically with most of the care providers who require data so that care coordination and patient safety can be implemented accurately. HIE programs contain mechanisms that are allowed to share most health information without any patient direct control and supervision. In this situation, many security issues and privacy risks may arise, and the patient's trust is very important as per HIE. The reactions obtained from patients can be thoroughly predicted based on the faith in the technology to seek assurance over the HIE networks without threatening personal health information or mishandling sensitive medical records before disclosing the information.

The distinct trust obtained in HIE models is based on the belief of distributed mechanisms with varying competence and integrity, as the patient HIE competency tends to determine the level of reliance on HIE technology to attain competent performance and efficiently transfer health information to a wide range of health institutions. The faith in HIE tends to integrate the notion of agreement between HIE patients who are trustworthy, as the distance acquired among distinct patients with definite users lacks direct interaction between various patients in HIE models. The centralized control that is exercised in healthcare organizations is unfamiliar when dealing with mechanisms that are used by the HIE system to share medical records electronically with factors that contribute towards a lack of trust. Almost all of the characteristics produce a more ethereal environment that performs tasks using traditional sharing methods like fax or mail, and there are aforementioned motives that may make patients confident, as it is more critical to exchange applied modifications using common methods such as direct, query-based and patient-mediated communication.

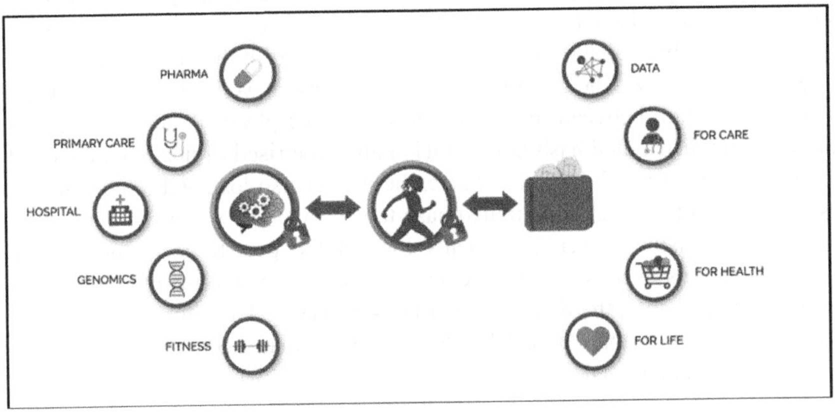

Figure 6.3. *Healthcare Blockchain*

HIE programs aim to build inter-organizational networks where a patient's medical records are shared over a number of geographically distant healthcare organizations, containing sensitive data that is shared through a networked-based technology, as there are privacy issues that are virtually worsened, and patient privacy has an impact on the accuracy of completeness with HIE patient databases. Most of the results are lost as there are ineffective therapies consisting of erroneous care planning with maximum mortality rates, and HIE networks must guarantee patients that their medical records are kept secure through the interchange process, based on the privacy policies readily available to highlight how sensitive health information in an organization is accessible by providing unauthorized access and secondary usage.

6.4.3.1. *Alternative for Blockchain-based HIE*

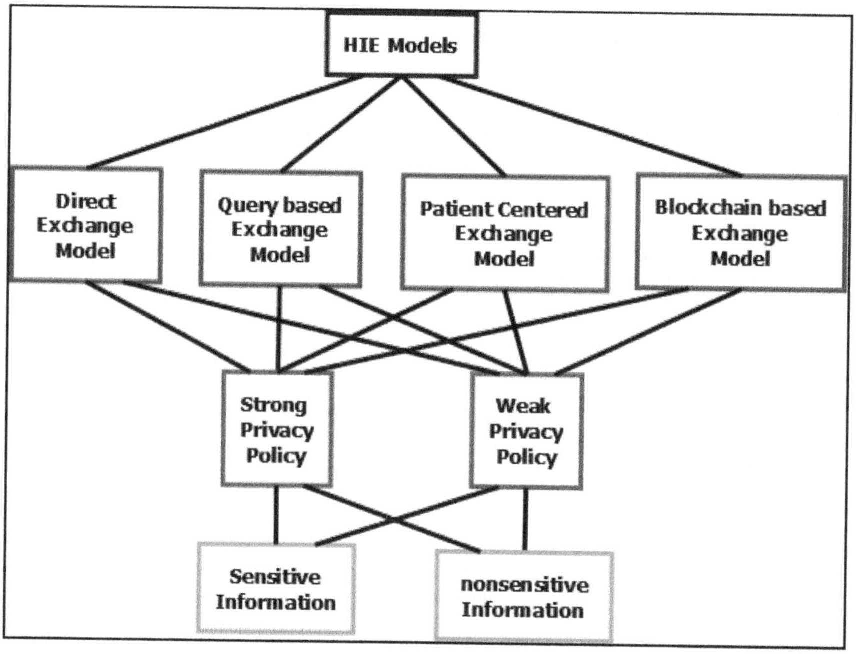

Figure 6.4. *HIE model*

Blockchain technology is increasing in popularity as it is a novel process of managing the business along with the commercial transactions by dynamically sharing the ledgers. Blockchain can make it easier to record economic transactions among parties that are involved directly or indirectly. In addition, because Blockchain is based on a peer-to-peer network of distinct nodes, it must eradicate the need for intermediary transactions and direct third-party control over a company's operations. The majority of Blockchain research has focused on the technological aspects of cryptocurrency. Blockchain technology, on the contrary, has a broader and deeper set of applications than virtual currencies, and can be used for more than just various economic transactions. The interest in Blockchain has risen by attracting a lot of attention and financing from a number of efforts across multiple industries. Blockchain technology is transforming almost all of the sectors and healthcare. Because of its foundation technology, one of the most acceptable processes of Blockchain is the development of trust in coordination and coordinating communication across networked businesses (such as hospitals).

Other organizational activities, such as the transmission of information between connected and unaffiliated healthcare firms, could benefit from Blockchain technology (parties involved or related to healthcare procedure or doctors or hospitals or clinics). It has been suggested that a Blockchain centered allotment of models takes advantage of the Blockchain's immutability and inherent autonomy, and can effectively track records to access the sensitive medical data that is deposited in the cloud. Blockchain-based admittance control architecture has the potential to help healthcare organizations that facilitate medical data allocation with distinct establishments.

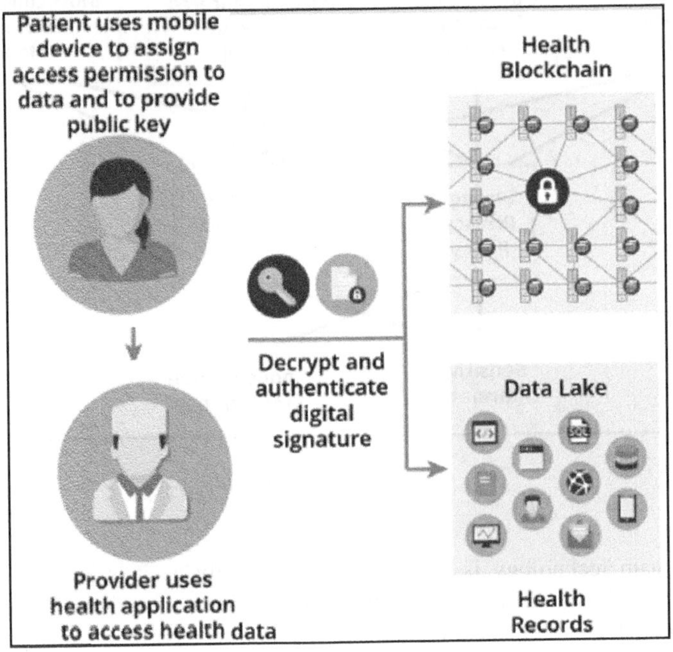

Figure 6.5. *Process of the model*

This technology consists of various protected cryptographic algorithms that are strictly controlled to access the patient medical records that are deposited and processed over cloud platforms. The sophisticated safety implemented in system architecture has the potential to detect and validate various users who tend to access critical medical records by keeping track of various sharing implementations.

6.5. Conclusion and future scope

In this chapter, Blockchain technology solves the interoperability problems based on the open standards that provide a shared distributed interpretation of healthcare data and is expected to be widely adopted and used across all health-related industries. Based on the proposed health Blockchain outlined in this study, most of the healthcare contributors and institutions, along with medical researchers, enlighten their research by imparting huge volumes of genetic, nutritional, lifestyle, environmental or healthcare data with guaranteed confidentiality and anonymity. HIE networks need to reassure patients with medical records that they are kept secure during the interchange process as per the privacy policies that emphasize sensitive health information to be used only in their treatment towards better health and disease prevention. Before creating an industry-ready solution, more work is required in strategic areas, as there are increased costs and incentives to implement data security and intellectual property preservation.

6.6. References

Ahram, T., Sargolzaci, A., Sargolzaei, S., Daniels, J., Amaba, B. (2017). Blockchain technology innovations. *IEEE Technology & Engineering Management Conference (TEMSCON)*, 137–141.

Ahsan, M.M., Wahab, A.W.A., Idris, M.Y.I., Khan, S., Bachura, E., Choo, K.-K.R. (2020). CLASS: Cloud log assuring soundness and secrecy scheme for cloud forensics. *IEEE Trans. Sustain. Comput.*, 6(2), 184–196.

Al Omar, A., Rahman, M.S., Basu, A., Kiyomoto, S. (2017). Medibchain: A blockchain based privacy preserving platform for healthcare data. *International Conference on Security, Privacy and Anonymity in Computation, Communication and Storage*, 534–543. Springer.

Azaria, A., Ekblaw, A., Vieira, T., Lippman, A. (2016). Medrec: Using blockchain for medical data access and permission management. *2nd International Conference on Open and Big Data (OBD), IEEE*, 25–30.

Bahga, A. and Madisetti, V.K. (2013). A cloud-based approach for interoperable electronic health records (EHRs). *IEEE J. Biomed. Health Inform.*, 17(5), 894–906.

Begoyan, A. (2007). An overview of interoperability standards for electronic health records. *USA Society for Design and Process Science*.

Benchoufi, M. and Ravaud, P. (2017). Blockchain technology for improving clinical research quality. *Trials*, 18(1), 335.

Blum, M., Feldman, P., Micali, S. (1988). Non-interactive zero-knowledge and its applications (extended abstract). *Proceedings of the 20th Annual ACM Symposium on Theory of Computing*, 2–4 May, Chicago, IL.

Boonstra, A., Versluis, A., Vos, J.F. (2014). Implementing electronic health records in hospitals: A systematic literature review. *BMC Health Serv. Res.*, 14(1), 370.

Carvalho, J.V., Rocha, Á., Abreu, A. (2016). Maturity models of healthcare information systems and technologies: A literature review. *J. Med. Syst.*, 40(6), 131.

Castro, M. and Liskov, B. (1999). Practical Byzantine fault tolerance. *Symposium on Operating Systems Design & Implementation*, New Orleans, LA.

Crameri, K.-A., Maher, L., Van Dam, P., Prior, S. (2020). Personal electronic healthcare records: What influences consumers to engage with their clinical data online? A literature review. *Health Inf. Manag. J.*, 1833358319895369.

Daemen, J. and Rijmen, V. (2002). *The Design of Rijndael: AES – The Advanced Encryption Standard*. Springer, Berlin, Heidelberg.

Dai, W., Dai, C., Choo, K.R., Cui, C., Zou, D., Jin, H. (2020). SDTE: A secure Blockchain-based data trading ecosystem. *IEEE Trans. Inf. Forens. Secur.*, 15, 725–737.

Dias, J.P., Reis, L., Ferreira, H.S., Martins, Â. (2018). Blockchain for access control in e-health scenarios. arXiv:1805.12267.

Esposito, C., Santis, A.D., Tortora, G., Chang, H., Choo, K.R. (2018). Blockchain: A panacea for healthcare cloud-based data security and privacy? *IEEE Cloud Comput.*, 5(1), 3137.

Ethereum (n.d.). Ethereum [Online]. Available at: https://www.ethereum.org/.

Feng, Q., He, D., Liu, Z., Wang, D., Choo, K.-K.R. (2020). Multi-party signing protocol for the identity-based signature scheme in IEEE p1363 standard. *IET Information Security*, 1(99), 1–10. DOI: 10.1049/iet-ifs.2019.0559.

Kumar, R.R., Reddy, B., Pappula, P. (2019). An evaluation of feature selection algorithms in machine learning. *International Journal of Scientific & Technology Research*, 8(12), 2071–2074.

Praveen, P. and Jayanth Babu, C. (2019). Big data clustering: Applying conventional data mining techniques in big data environment. *Innovations in Computer Science and Engineering, Lecture Notes in Networks and Systems*, 74. DOI: 10.1007/978-981-13-7082-3_58.

Praveen, P., Shaik, M.A., Kumar, T.S., Choudhury, T. (2021). Smart farming: Securing farmers using block chain technology and IOT. In *Blockchain Applications in IoT Ecosystem*, Choudhury, T., Khanna, A., Toe, T.T., Khurana, M., Gia Nhu, N. (eds). Springer, Cham. DOI: 10.1007/978-3-030-65691-1_15.

Rama, B., Praveen, P., Sinha, H., Choudhury, T. (2017). A study on causal rule discovery with PC algorithm. *2017 International Conference on Infocom Technologies and Unmanned Systems (Trends and Future Directions) (ICTUS)*, Dubai, 616–621. DOI: 10.1109/ICTUS.2017.8286083.

7

Patient Data Privacy Using Blockchain

With rapid transformation in the healthcare industry, the enablement of Information Technology and digitalization of healthcare services has increased the use of electronic health records (EHRs) exponentially. On one side of a coin this has many advantages like enhancing patient care, more efficient record management, research advancement, etc., but the other side of the coin warns us about the complexity in maintaining anonymity of patient data and being compliant to the privacy laws and regulations. The interest of hackers is already moving towards the healthcare industry, and there have been so many events in past few years where patient data in large amounts has been breached and misused. Healthcare entities are trying to protect patient data; still, there are so many breaches, the actual reason is that most of the controls are towards data security and there are many times when we may believe that security controls also safeguard privacy, but it is not true, and this generates the gap. Multiple data privacy laws and some laws/standards specific to healthcare data like Health Information Technology for Economic and Clinical Health (HITECH) Act of 2009, Health Insurance Portability and Accountability Act of 1996 (HIPAA), General Data Protection Regulation (GDPR), etc. provide various security and data privacy requirements which all healthcare entities need to comply with. These laws also provide various rights to the patients like consent, right to control, right to dispose, etc. Therefore, now the real question is how to implement data privacy controls which will maintain patient data anonymization, at the same time as making sure that healthcare entities comply with privacy laws and regulations and that all rights of the patients towards their data are also preserved: thus, the answer is Blockchain. The major features of Blockchain, i.e. decentralization, transparency and security make it a perfect fit for privacy protection. With the help of Blockchain, an environment can be created in which all patients can review their data before it becomes part of the records, permissioned Blockchain can solve the issue of patient data access and control, consensus algorithms and smart contracts will prevent patient data tampering and unauthorized access. It is known that bitcoins are pseudonymous, but with privacy preserving protocols for the Blockchain, it is possible to achieve anonymity. Similarly, one of the best things that Blockchain can provide for patient data privacy is its role as a data controller. The data controller and data processor are two important roles

---

For a color version of all figures in this chapter, see www.iste.co.uk/choudhury/blockchain.zip.

Chapter written by Jatin SETHI and ALIND.

defined in multiple laws defining data protection responsibilities, hence the implementation of Blockchain for data privacy can compensate the responsibilities of the data controller with better transparency. With the integration of Blockchain in healthcare services or in creating healthcare applications, we can achieve Privacy by Design.

7.1. Introduction

Well-being is the establishment of cheerful life, and the current generation has been the luckiest beneficiary of extraordinary advances in clinical innovation. With each innovation, more pieces of information become accessible to translate the issues that plague our prosperity. This information is highly sensitive as it is the Electronic Health Record (EHR). EHR is the sensitive private information of the patients which is usually shared between patients, clinics/hospitals, pharmaceuticals, health insurance companies, test laboratories, etc. The complex part is to track this data down with multiple entities storing and maintaining data. Healthcare interoperability is fixated on the trading of information, a wide accessible interoperability brings new difficulties and prerequisites with respect to security, anonymity and administration (Magyar 2018; Guimarães et al. 2020; Huang and Lee 2020).

There are four main concerned areas that address the challenges in EHR management (Engelhardt 2017; Rejeb et al. 2021):

a) Patient-centric: usually patients interact with a variety of healthcare entities and provide their data to multiple EHR management tools. This procedure increases the agreement that all data at different entities shall be available to the patient all of the time, so that the patient can take control of their information and access it at anytime.

b) Data privacy: EHR being sensitive personal data demands privacy and accessible only by authorized parties at appropriate times. This is still a rather complex area since there are many laws and regulations which mandate different principles of data privacy to be in place in the form of privacy controls by the entities which collect, process or transmit healthcare data.

c) Data integrity: data integrity is all about data completeness, consistency and accuracy. By ensuring that complete health information is available to the right people at the right time, patient-centric information exchange should give patients more control and better outcomes.

d) Cost: the health expenditure around the globe has increased in the past few decades; still, there is a crisis in healthcare costs. There have been many cases where lots of money has been put into EHR but has gone to waste due to there being less acceptance by people of a certain age group, especially for countries with an aging population. There have also been other factors like security issues, user friendliness and comfortability in using EHR, etc.

7.2. Threat modeling – digitalization in the healthcare industry

Digitalization in the healthcare industry is not only about digitalizing the core infrastructure, making healthcare instruments IT enabled or increasing automation/robotics in medical treatments/surgeries (Sharma et al. 2021), but also how this digitalization can be extended to the end-user is the major chunk of automation; however, extending digitalization to the end-user comes at its own cost, this cost is not only monetary but also balancing the fact that the end-user wants it to be as user-friendly, robust and reliable as possible, and at the same time the services/products need to be secured by its design (Singh and Talapula 2019). This means that while in digitalizing we cannot rely on the end-user for security, because that is the most vulnerable end, the services and products shall be developed with security by design principle, i.e. foundationally secure.

Around a decade back, digitalization from an end-user perspective was completely dependent on web applications which were accessible via computers, laptops, etc., but with recent advancements in smartphone technology, where smart mobile devices are available at lost costs, everything has changed. This now means that for the end-user, dependency on hardware requirements like a computer or laptop has vanished which has potentially increased the number of end-users who are willing to use healthcare applications via their mobile phones.

These mobile phones are smart because they not only provide end-users an application with a user-friendly interface to access their health records, chat over voice and video with doctors but they are also able to sense changes in temperature, human body measurements, etc. (Papageorgiou et al. 2018). Due to the advance processing capabilities of the smart phones, mobile applications not only provide a platform to store health records, but also have access to live locations and sensitive data like photographs, videos, contacts, etc.

Hence while using health applications, sensitive data is at stake, due to which all health application service providers need to follow many legal regulations and requirements to ensure data privacy and security. Therefore, the actual challenge is providing digitalized healthcare services and implementing security and privacy controls which are also aligned or suffice all legal requirements. To understand this better, in this section, we will take a generic example of a healthcare application, and will try to understand the flow of data, threat surface and possible attack scenarios.

The purpose of the two sections below is to first understand the foundations of data flow in healthcare and then to understand the real security challenges in the current system, so that once we move further and discuss security and privacy controls using Blockchain in the coming sections, we can easily correlate it with the problem statement.

7.2.1. *Data flow diagram (DFD)*

Healthcare applications may vary as per the type of service (i.e. online doctor consultation, ordering medicines online, pathological test, any hospital specific for their patients, etc.). Therefore, the detailed data flow will also vary as per the type of application and entities involved in it.

However, in this section, a generic example has been taken which will be same at high level for all types of healthcare applications. This DFD will be used further in this section to analyze threats and security controls. Figure 7.1 helps us to demonstrate a high-level DFD, which includes an end-user on the left who will access the application user interface by using either smart phones or their computers. Then, based on type of services, the user interaction will connect with the Health Application Service at service provider end. During this interaction, data will also flow bidirectionally. The middle part of this DFD, i.e. Health Application Service is the most complex part where all of the processing of data and storage of data will occur based on the type of application and its functionality, since this is high-level DFD, hence this part is shown in a box, otherwise this itself will actually have multiple layers like a web server, an application server, a database server, cloud services, etc. The lower the level on this part, the better and more detailed threat analysis will be.

The final part is also very important, i.e. with the involvement of third parties, as the market is growing, it has been noted that different application providers are collaborating to expand their business. Let us take an example, healthcare application HA1 whose main functionality was to provide an online consultation by doctors to the patients. Later on, HA1 decided to go into business with another company, and created HA2, whose functionality is to sell medicines online. Nowadays, HA2 is integrated on HA1 as a third party. So as soon as patient consultation is completed, the application HA1 tries to automatically redirect the patient to HA2 from their platform to make them buy medicines from HA2. This means that the patient does not need to create any data on HA2, but the application HA1 will transfer the patient's details and prescription to HA2 via an API. This whole process makes it very easy for the patient and business is increased for both parties, but at the same time, the question of security controls while transferring patient data to a third party also comes to mind. Not only this but also the question of privacy controls comes to mind because now there is a dependency on the third party which is accessing the sensitive personal data of the patient.

The flow of data is shown in Figure 7.1, and DFD has been shown by using the arrows.

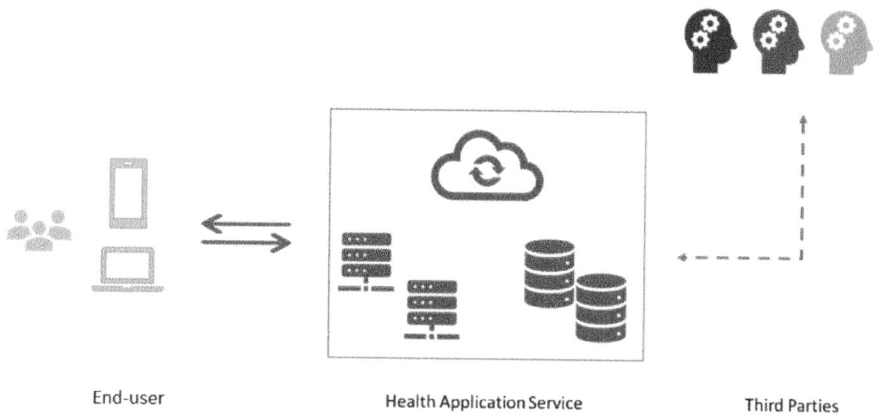

Figure 7.1. *A generic healthcare application – high-level DFD*

Now let us discuss the famous term "connected health" (Papageorgiou et al. 2018). With the increase in automation and digitalization of healthcare services, this is not only patient-centric but is also used across the healthcare industry. In the whole healthcare industry, there are various entities that are dependent on each other. The digitalization has been boon for all the entities as now they can connect with each other, the data collected/generated at one entity can be shared with other entity very easily, hence it is called "connected health", where the goal is to achieve a smart health paradigm. A simple example has been discussed above for the two applications HA1 and HA2.

Figure 7.2 shows a less complex demonstration of "connected health"; however, in reality, it may become more complex. The purpose here is to visualize and understand the depth of the security and privacy challenges because health records are being shared across so many entities. The high-level DFD shown in Figure 7.1 is for one entity, and Figure 7.2 can help us to understand that when this data flow is scaled in a connected health model, the complexity will also increase exponentially.

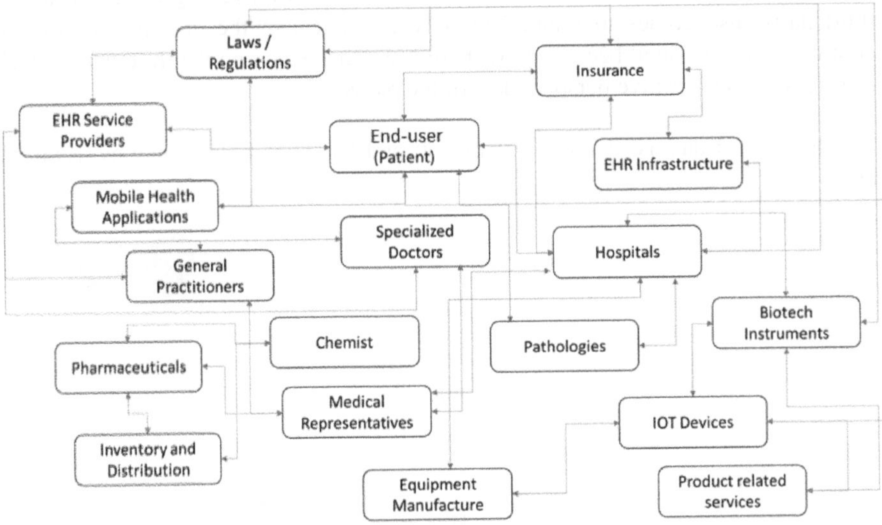

Figure 7.2. *Digitalization in healthcare industry – connected health and service model*

7.2.2. *Threat analysis*

In continuation to above discussed DFD in Figure 7.1, let us start with drawing threat surfaces on it. Firstly, let us understand threat surfaces: these are set of points in a complete system where the attacker can try to exploit vulnerabilities. Figure 7.3 helps us to identify threat surfaces in the high-level DFD as discussed above; all the attack surfaces are represented in dotted ovals/circles.

These attack surfaces can be broken into various vulnerabilities and possible attacks based on their locations like DoS, spoofing, man in middle, sniffing or tampering of data, etc. Let us elaborate on the attack surfaces and understand them with some examples as shown in Figure 7.1.

Always remember, the lower the level of DFD, the better and more detailed the threat analysis.

S. no.	Attack surface	Attack scenarios (threat–vulnerability pairing)
1	AS1	Use of outdated/unpatched operating systems in end-user devices
2	AS1	Unauthorized access of non-required pictured, i.e. privilege escalation by healthcare application
3	AS2	Man in the middle attack like packet sniffing
4	AS2	Man in the middle attack like session hijacking
5	AS3	Denial of service (DoS)/distributed denial of service (DDoS) attack on servers
6	AS3	Vulnerabilities in code of application may help attacker in tampering the services, erasing everything, etc.
7	AS3	Unpatched servers/security misconfiguration may help attackers in gaining unauthorized remote access of the servers
8	AS3	Insufficient logging and monitoring
9	AS4	Unauthorized access of sensitive data by third-party applications
10	AS4	Man in the middle attack-like packet sniffing

Table 7.1. *Threat analysis for DFD shown in Figures 7.1 and 7.2*

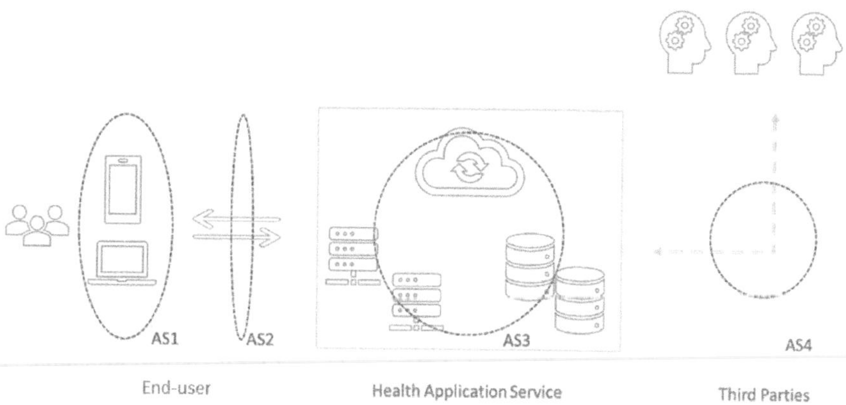

Figure 7.3. *Threat surfaces mapping in a generic health application – high-level DFD*

7.3. Privacy versus security

Before moving further, it is important to understand the difference between security and privacy. This is important because in many organizations and with many security engineers/managers, it has been observed that once security controls are implemented, it is considered that privacy would be taken care of too; however, this is not the case. People get confused because they use both the words interchangeably and consider both means data protection; however, the truth is that security and privacy are different yet have similar components which creates ambiguity.

Information security is about preservation of confidentiality, integrity and availability. The meaning of confidentiality is to keep data safe from unauthorized access, integrity means preserving the accuracy of data and keeping it reliable, and availability means that data should be accessible by authorized users/services whenever required. However, privacy starts from the control of collection of personal data, the control of use of personal data and goes as far as the control of destruction/disposal of data.

It is important to understand that security can be achieved without privacy, but privacy cannot be achieved without security. Security controls focus on all information while privacy controls focus on PII, i.e. personally identifiable information, personal data or sensitive personal data.

To keep it simple, security preserves integrity, confidentiality and availability of data while privacy preserves the protection of privacy rights with respect to the processing of data and data anonymity.

7.3.1. *Privacy in Blockchain*

Before getting into privacy in Blockchain, let us recall some basic terminologies. A distributed ledger is a kind of database which is spread across various computer devices usually in different geographical locations. Distributed ledger technology is the name given to any technology which helps in storing and updating the distributed ledger (Belotti et al. 2019; Ul Hassan et al. 2020). Blockchain is a distributed ledger system that allows for the sharing of a validated ledger of transactions which are kept in blocks and connected by a chain. The genesis block is the very first block on the Blockchain, and all subsequent blocks are added sequentially onto it. Privacy in Blockchain is achieved by three key principles, i.e. cryptography, decentralization and consensus algorithm (Tian et al. 2019; Sharma and Balamurugan 2020):

– **Cryptography:** hashing is a well-known cryptography terminology; hashing is a mathematical function that creates a value of specific size for any data in this case block, and if there is any change in this data (block), the hash value will change. This means that the hash value assures the integrity of data (block). Each block on a Blockchain contains the hash of the previous block, and along with the hash, each block also consists of a timestamp, a nonce and a record, i.e. transaction data. In the term Blockchain, chain is the hash value because it is a reference to the prior block for each block. Figure 7.4 shows a representation of how blocks are connected and referee previous blocks with the help of hash values.

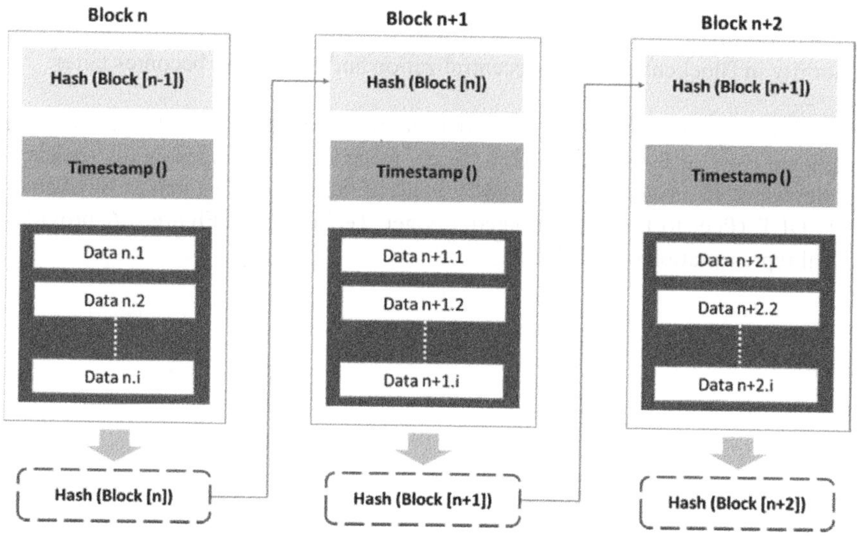

Figure 7.4. *Blockchain structure*

Another well-known terminology in the world of cryptography is digital signature. Every participant in the network has their own private key which they use for signing the block, i.e. creation of a digital signature for every block. Figure 7.5 demonstrates the traditional workings of digital signatures.

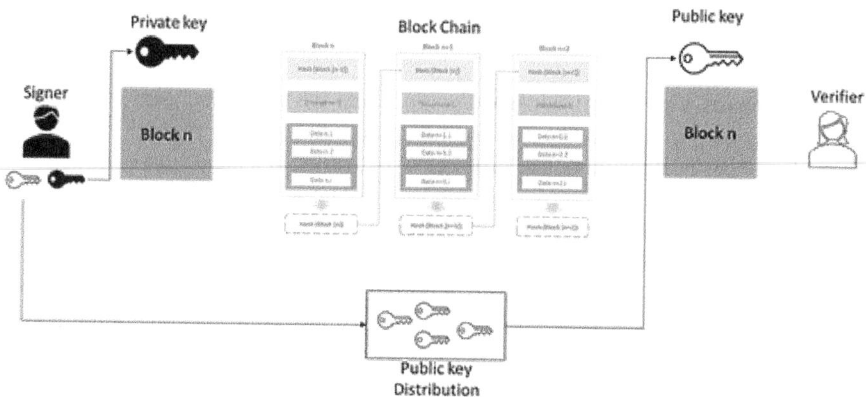

Figure 7.5. *Working of digital signature*

– **Decentralization:** with the help of digital signature, it is clear that if there is any alteration with the block, then the digital signature will become illegal and the peers in the network will be informed that manipulation has occurred. This whole process becomes more efficient with decentralization as there will be no single authority in Blockchain during decentralization and the system becomes fairer.

The beauty of decentralization is that no node can manipulate ledger but have a duplicate copy of ledger with them, hence, to make any changes in any transaction in the ledger a consensus is required from all of the nodes. This makes Blockchain a P2P DLT (Peer-to-Peer, Distributed Ledger Technology). Figure 7.6 provides a visual representation of P2P DLT.

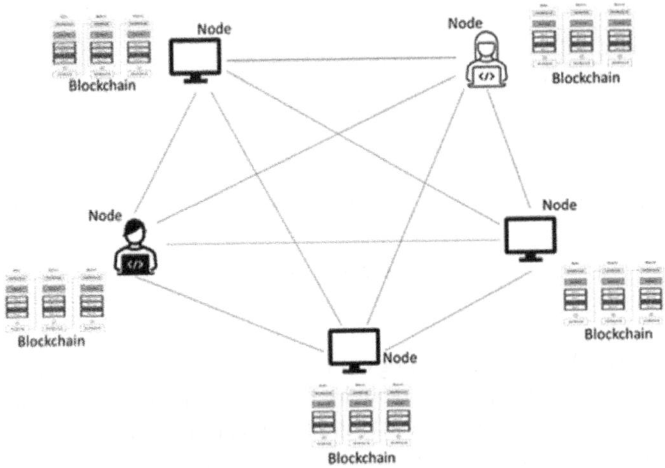

Figure 7.6. *Blockchain – a P2P DLT*

– **Consensus algorithm:** consensus algorithms have already been discussed in previous chapters in detail. The purpose here is not to again go through all different types of consensus algorithms like proof of work, proof of state, smart contracts, etc. but to understand how consensus algorithms help in preserving privacy in Blockchain. During our discussion in section 7.3, it was clear that privacy is also about protection of rights (privacy rights) and consensus algorithms, thus this helps in that part. The purpose of consensus algorithms is to ensure data in the ledger is same for all the nodes, and every node agrees to a process of achieving the correct state of the data which means there is an agreement between all of the nodes. This agreement varies based on the functionality and purpose of the Blockchain.

To correlate with a real-life example, consensus algorithms can be compared to a data privacy regulation/law that mandates all the parties to adhere to some of the principles for the preservation of data privacy.

7.3.2. *Process flow*

Let us take some examples to understand the process flow of healthcare applications using Blockchain technology (Li et al. 2018; Belotti et al. 2019; Clim and Zota 2019; Usman and Qamar 2020; Dash et al. 2021). Here, we will consider different types of healthcare applications and explain their system when the same application is designed using Blockchain technology.

The first example is a straightforward online consultation healthcare application which is used by patients to consult with their doctors online via a healthcare portal; let's name it HealthConsult for reference. Considering HealthConsult is developed using Blockchain technology, the high-level architecture is visualized in Figure 7.7. Figure 7.7 simply shows that Blockchain is used in this application, while Figure 7.8 shows a more detailed low-level architecture that clearly explains the process flow of how interactions will occur between a patient and a doctor via Blockchain. An important aspect of privacy and security is to understand that this Blockchain will be a permissioned Blockchain, i.e. only registered nodes in the network can access or append records in the Blockchain. Other than the permissioned Blockchain, it will have all of the standard features of Blockchain, i.e. hashing, digital signature, encryption, decentralization, consensus algorithm and smart contracts.

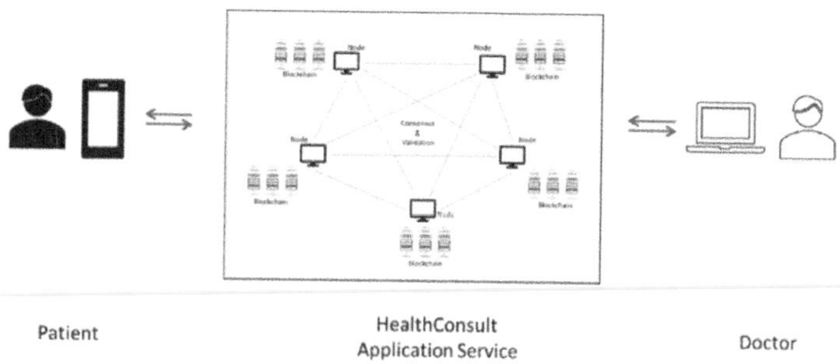

Figure 7.7. *Process flow – Example 1 (high-level architecture)*

Let us take another example, consider there is a hospital HP1 which has its own private Blockchain for the patients being treated there. HP1 store its patients' data in the private Blockchain. Now consider the scenario where a patient is referred to another hospital and say HP2 and HP2 want to access the patient data to see the history of the patient before starting any treatment. It is possible to provide data to a third party, i.e. HP2 in this case, but what we need to understand here is that data sharing is not manual via email or physical documents. Instead, we here consider a scenario where an IT-enabled system at HP2 will connect with systems at HP1 and after proper validation, it will access the data. However, in this whole process, there are lot of security challenges such as unauthorized access, elevation of privileges, man in the middle attacks, data leakage, etc. Security controls need to be implemented, some at the perimeter level, and some at the code level too to remediate different security threats, but this will make the system too complex. The consortium Blockchain is the solution here, meaning that there will be a network of hospitals. Every hospital will have their own private Blockchains, and at the same time, a permissioned Blockchain will be created which will be managed by authorized hospitals of the network, this Blockchain is also known as the consortium Blockchain. All hospitals can access the consortium Blockchain using a search index and can look for patient records. Figure 7.9 provides a visualization of this example. It is important to understand that Figure 7.9 is high level; moreover, the low-level architecture will provide the workings of the consensus mechanism, Blockchain-based sharing, the workings of the search index and most importantly validation of requests.

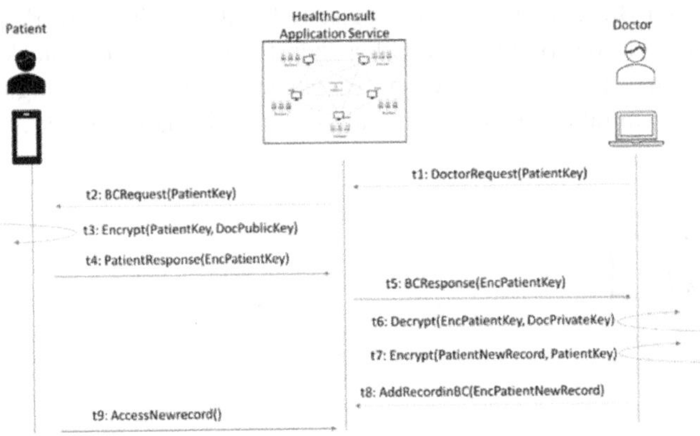

Figure 7.8. *Process flow – Example 1 (low-level architecture)*

We have just learned in the last example how multiple hospitals can connect with the help of a consortium Blockchain. Similarly, different health institutions can train a disease classification model collaboratively. This is possible using permissioned Blockchain which will use centralized distributed machine learning to train the model collaboratively, where every hospital will use their own patients' health records. During this training, every healthcare institution will first use inner calculations which will be followed by cross institution aggregation. This type of work has been proposed in various research lately in the name of health-chain, trained health-chain, etc. as this model is privacy preserving and allows healthcare institutions to train disease model collaboratively with a wide range of datasets (Chen et al. 2018, 2019; Li et al. 2018).

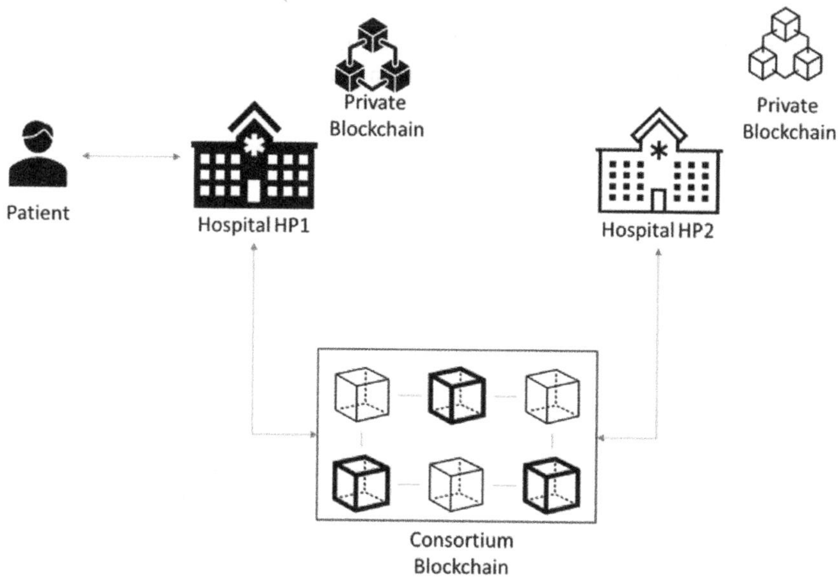

Figure 7.9. *Process flow – Example 2*

7.4. Regulatory compliance requirements

With the increase in size of data along with emerging technologies such as IoT, cloud, big data, etc., the instances of data breach have also increased. The impact of any data breach is very high when it involves sensitive data like health records. PHI (protected health information) suffers from a greater risk. In the last decade, there have been many cases of PHI breaches either by hospital electronic health record management systems or by insurance service providers, or by mobile healthcare applications such as online doctor consultations, online medicine buying apps, etc. Hence to strengthen medical data privacy and security governance, many countries have come up with regulations like HIPAA, HITECH, etc., even GDPR (General Data Protection Regulation) is not specifically for medical data, but it covers general data which means that any medical data breach in EU is also in the scope of GDPR (Jin et al. 2019).

7.4.1. *HIPAA, HITRUST, HITECH and GDPR (Shu and Jahankhani 2017; Magyar 2018; Jin et al. 2019)*

HIPAA is a US regulated act which is an abbreviation for the Health Insurance Portability and Accountability Act. HIPAA came into force in 1996 and since then there have been the following four major amendments:

– the Security Rule Amendment of 2003:

  - technical safeguards,

  - physical safeguards,

  - administrative safeguards;

– the Privacy Rule Amendment of 2003;

– the Breach Notification Rule of 2009;

– the Final Omnibus Rule of 2013.

In this section, we will cover the first three amendments (except physical and administrative, as that is not relevant to this chapter) because we are here trying to understand how Blockchain as a technology is helpful in compliance with regulatory requirements while the fourth amendment is related to business associates affected by HIPAA. So before jumping to the part concerning how Blockchain is helpful in compliance with regulatory requirements, let us first start with understanding the technical requirements that are part of the first three amendments. To keep it simple, Figure 7.10 can be used to visualize the outline of these requirements.

On the contrary, HITRUST is a privately held company which has developed a global security and privacy framework named HITRUST CSF in collaboration with healthcare, technology and information security organizations. HITRUST was originally an acronym for Health Information Trust Alliance.

HITECH Act is US based and its purpose is to enforce HIPAA security and privacy rules, and to encourage healthcare service providers for the adoption of EHR.

GDPR is also known as EU-GDPR which is an acronym for European General Data Protection Regulation, a regulation in Europe for data protection and privacy. However, GDPR has strengthened patient rights against their PHI and at the same time has increased security and privacy requirements for healthcare entities to protect PHI.

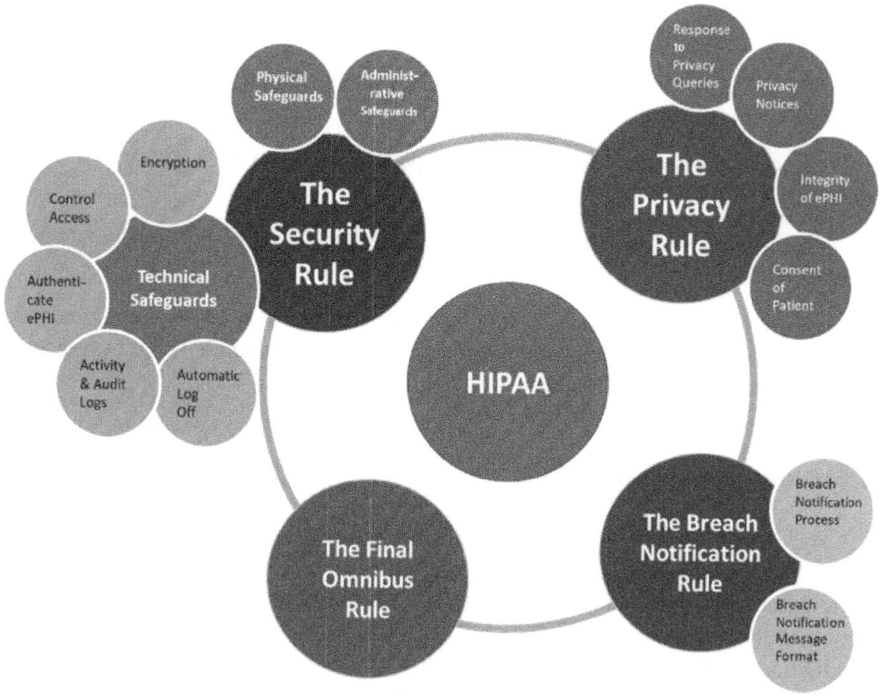

Figure 7.10. *HIPAA requirements*

7.4.2. *Blockchain as a savior*

The fundamental pillars of Blockchain can support security/privacy controls when different regulatory requirements need to be implemented in the form of technical controls (Yue et al. 2016; Kuo et al. 2017; Shu and Jahankhani 2017; Jin et al. 2019):

– Let us start with decentralization. In traditional healthcare applications DBMS is used while Blockchain provides decentralization which makes different healthcare entities collaborate without any central management entity. This is not possible so easily with DBMS.

– With the help of Blockchain, the PHI is more secure from any tampering as the ledger cannot be altered as Blockchain only supports the creation and reading of the ledgers.

– In Blockchain due to cryptography and digital signature, all records are digitally signed by the source hence all records are source verifiable.

– Due to decentralization, as data is not with a single node, it can never suffer a single point of failure issues, this makes data always available.

– As every block is encrypted in Blockchain by default, it makes sure that the confidentiality of data is not hampered.

– Blockchain enables and strengthens patient rights to own, share and control their data.

– Permissioned Blockchain assures that malicious nodes cannot participate in the network.

– Most importantly, many regulatory requirements related to compliance and agreement between the healthcare entity and patient can be implemented using smart contracts and consensus algorithms.

7.5. Differential privacy

The idea of differential privacy (Ul Hassan et al. 2020) was first introduced by C. Dwork in 2006 for statistical datasets. To understand it mathematically, differential privacy is adding noise in the data to preserve its privacy. Consider a function that analyzes a dataset and computes statistical results such as mean, median and variance. Now, if the algorithm of this function is enhanced in such a way that by looking at the output no one can tell whether an individual's data was used as input in the dataset or not, in this situation, the algorithm will be considered as differentially private (Ul Hassan et al. 2020).

Let us take a simple example: during market research, a team wants to know "how many people have watched the series Friends", "how many have watched Suits" and "how many have not watched Joker". Now if the system answering these questions have algorithms which are differentially private, it will first add noise to the real values and then will provide the approximate data to the market research team. This approximate data will draw the same conclusions as what actual data would have done so in this way it will not affect the market research team too. This is the main benefit of differential privacy, i.e. the data can be used for analysis while guaranteeing the protection of individual's privacy.

Let us take another example: a curator asks a medical data owner to check a dataset of patients who have died in the last five years in a particular city and answer for each patient whether they died of cancer. The medical data owner agrees to provide an approximate count based on an algorithm, rather giving actual data. The algorithm has been visualized in Figure 7.11. For each patient row, firstly the medical data owner will flip a coin, if it turns to be heads, then they will tell the truth to the curator. Yet if turns to be "tails", then they will again flip a coin, now if it is "heads", then they will answer "yes" and if it is "tails", then they will answer "no" to the curator. In this way as per probability, the curator will know the truth almost half of the time, and for other half, there will be a random answer that will also have some "truth", so the curator will have an approximate answer.

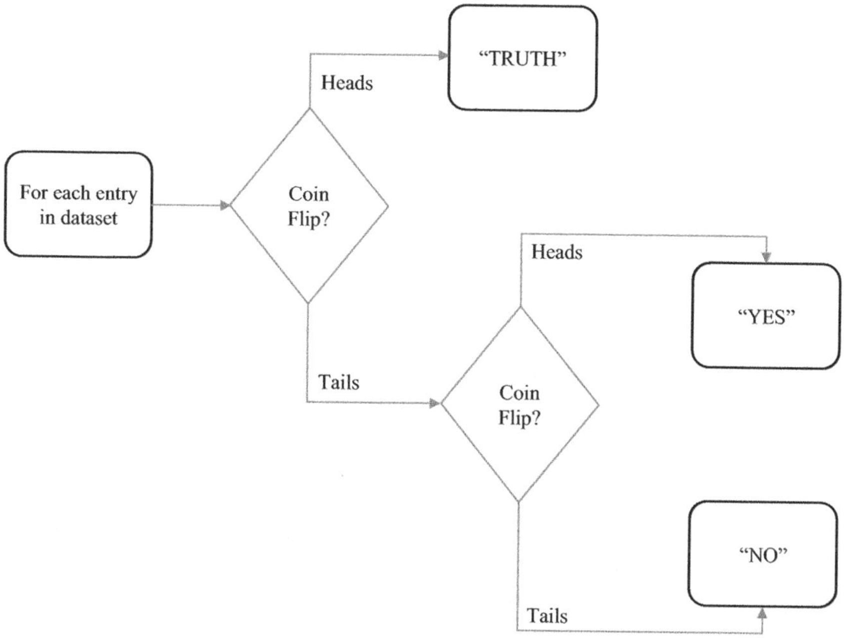

Figure 7.11. *Differential privacy algorithm example*

7.5.1. *Local differential privacy versus global differential privacy (Ul Hassan et al. 2020)*

Consider a scenario where a researcher requests some kind of data for analysis to multiple data generators. In the local private system, each data generator will generate raw data, add noise to it and send data to the researcher. While in global privacy system, each data generator will firstly send data to a trusted curator, who will aggregate the data (or group the data), then add noise to it and provide it to the researcher. These two systems are shown in Figure 7.12.

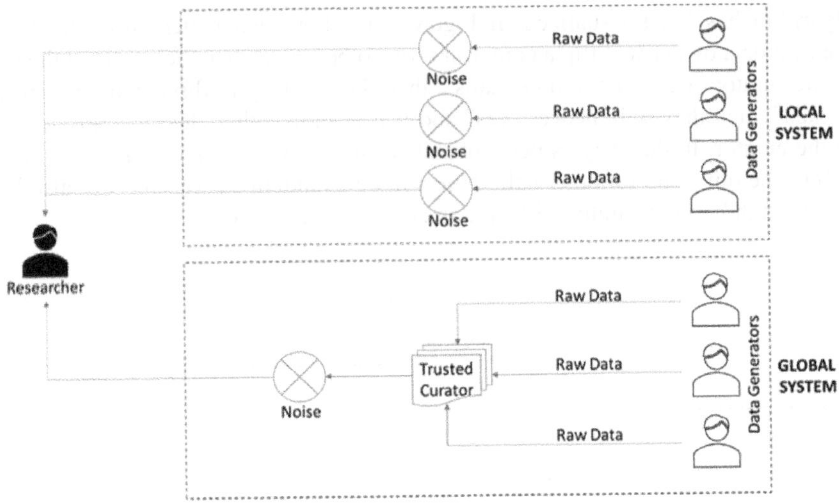

Figure 7.12. *Local system and global system*

7.5.2. *Quantification of privacy and mathematical form of differential privacy (Sun et al. 2019; Ul Hassan et al. 2020)*

Differential privacy quantifies privacy. It does not define privacy as a binary value, for example if data has been or has not been leaked, but quantifies privacy as "privacy loss" which is at risk of being exposed. The value for "privacy loss" will increase with the number of times data is processed. The terms, which are used in equation [7.1], are given as follows:

– the parameter ε represents the privacy loss;

– D1 and D2 represent the adjacent dataset;

– F is the randomized function for differential privacy and the range of F is D1 x D2;

– P is the probability which satisfies if and only if (O ∈ F), where O is the output of F. We obtain the following:

$$P[F(D1) \in O] \leq \exp(\varepsilon) \times P[F(D2) \in O] \qquad [7.1]$$

In this case, Range(F) is the maximum value for the function F and ε is the parameter for privacy loss which helps in controlling the privacy level.

7.5.3. *Advantages of using differential privacy in Blockchain*

Now as we have already explained the concept of differential privacy, it will be easier to understand how it is useful in Blockchain. The fundamental features of Blockchain, which make it the next generation of secured storage, and using differential privacy in Blockchain will enhance the privacy of Blockchain. Some examples are given below:

– protection of sender and receiver addresses from punitive and feather forking attacks, and linking attacks;

– protecting network-wide privacy from a deanonymization attack;

– preserving data during consensus;

– protection from a trinity attack.

7.6. Privacy by Design

Privacy by Design and Privacy by Default are frequently used terminologies, especially since new privacy regulations started coming into the picture. Privacy by Design aims to integrate privacy requirements and controls in all new systems where personal information is in scope. This means Privacy by Design recommends that from the very start of a product/system development, privacy requirements shall be considered and shall be integrated in the design and architecture of the system, so that when a system is developed, all privacy controls are embedded in the system. On the other hand, Privacy by Default talks about post development, i.e. privacy settings shall be enabled by default once a product/system is deployed in production.

The concept of Privacy by Design was first discussed by the former Canadian Information and Privacy Commissioner Ann Cavoukian, as she created several principles as foundation of Privacy by Design. The purpose of these principles is to make privacy integral to priorities of the organization, project objectives and design process. The seven principles of Privacy by Design are discussed (Kurtz et al. 2018; Romanou 2018; Wahlstrom et al. 2020) in Figure 7.13.

From the Blockchain point of view, many of these principles can be easily followed because of the fundamental features of the Blockchain. However, it is highly recommended while creating any system/application using Blockchain to first list all privacy requirements and then create a map that will be automatically sufficed by Blockchain features, the one that needs to be covered in consensus algorithms and smart contracts, and finally the one that needs addon security/privacy features to be integrated into Blockchain to enhance its security and privacy capabilities such as differential privacy and proxy re-encryption.

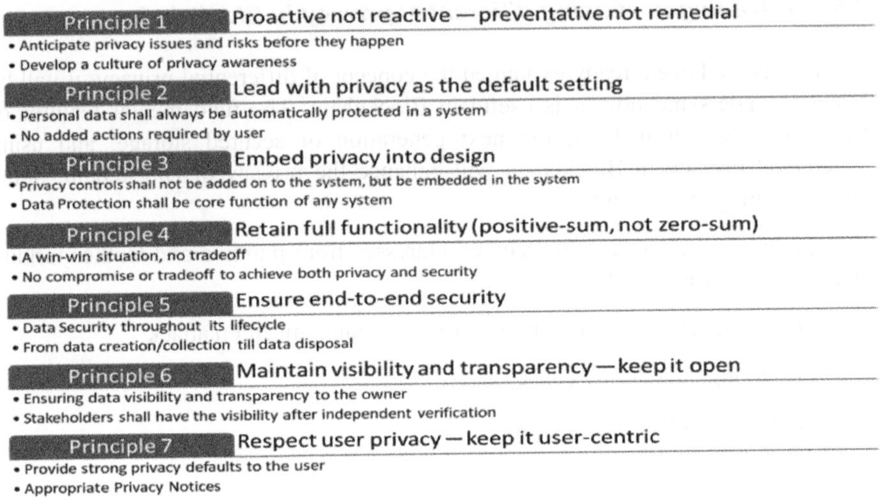

Figure 7.13. *Privacy by Design principles*

7.7. Conclusion

Blockchain technology has been considered a game changer and that is why industries like banking are adopting it for faster transactions, cost reduction, improving security and record keeping. In the healthcare industry, Blockchain can become a valuable generating factor for healthcare entities because it can allow different healthcare entities to share their networks without compromising data security and integrity yet will still allow for them to track the source and the changes. With increased digitalization in the healthcare domain, trust has gained importance along with security and Blockchain because of its fundamental principles which provide trust, security and privacy. With the involvement of IoT in healthcare, the interdependency has increased following the need of security during communication, which has also increased. Now, the need of the hour is more research on developing prototypes of healthcare applications based on the type of services using Blockchain as backbone. This will help in scaling Blockchain in the healthcare domain.

7.8. References

Belotti, M., Božić, N., Pujolle, G., Secci, S. (2019). A vademecum on Blockchain technologies: When, which, and how. *IEEE Commun. Surv. Tutorials*, 21, 3796–3838. DOI: 10.1109/COMST.2019.2928178.

Chen, Y., Ding, S., Xu, Z., Zheng, H., Yang, S. (2018). Blockchain-based medical records secure storage and medical service framework. *J. Med. Syst.*, 43. DOI: 10.1007/s10916-018-1121-4.

Chen, X., Wang, X., Yang, K. (2019). Asynchronous Blockchain-based privacy-preserving training framework for disease diagnosis. *2019 IEEE International Conference on Big Data (Big Data)*, 5469–5473. DOI: 10.1109/BigData47090.2019.9006173.

Clim, A., Zota, R.D., Constantinescu, R. (2019). Data exchanges based on Blockchain in m-health applications. *Procedia Comput. Sci.*, 160, 281–288. DOI: 10.1016/j.procs.2019.11.088.

Dash, S., Gantayat, P.K., Das, R.K. (2021). Blockchain technology in healthcare: Opportunities and challenges. In *Intelligent Systems Reference Library*, Panda, S.K., Jena, A.K., Swain, S.K., Satapathy, S.C. (eds). Springer International Publishing, Cham. DOI: 10.1007/978-3-030-69395-4_6.

Engelhardt, M.A. (2017). Hitching healthcare to the chain: An introduction to Blockchain technology in the healthcare sector. *Technol. Innov. Manag. Rev.*, 7, 22–34. DOI: 10.22215/timreview/1111.

Guimarães, T., Silva, H., Peixoto, H., Santos, M. (2020). Modular Blockchain implementation in intensive medicine. *Procedia Comput. Sci.*, 170, 1059–1064. DOI: 10.1016/j.procs.2020.03.073.

Huang, L. and Lee, H.H. (2020). A medical data privacy protection scheme based on Blockchain and cloud computing. *Wireless Communications and Mobile Computing*, 8859961. DOI: 10.1155/2020/8859961.

Jin, H., Luo, Y., Li, P., Mathew, J. (2019). A review of secure and privacy-preserving medical data sharing. *IEEE Access.*, 7, 61656–61669. DOI: 10.1109/ACCESS.2019.2916503.

Kuo, T.T., Kim, H.E., Ohno-Machado, L. (2017). Blockchain distributed ledger technologies for biomedical and health care applications. *J. Am. Med. Informatics Assoc.*, 24, 1211–1220. DOI: 10.1093/jamia/ocx068.

Kurtz, C., Semmann, M., Böhmann, T. (2018). Privacy by design to comply with GDPR: A review on third-party data processors. *Am. Conf. Inf. Syst.*, Digit. Disruption, AMCIS, 1–10.

Li, H., Zhu, L., Shen, M., Gao, F., Tao, X., Liu, S. (2018). Blockchain-based data preservation system for medical data. *J. Med. Syst.*, 42, 1–13. DOI: 10.1007/s10916-018-0997-3.

Magyar, G. (2017). Blockchain: Solving the privacy and research availability tradeoff for EHR data: A new disruptive technology in health data management. *IEEE 30th Jubil. Neumann Colloquium*, 135–140. DOI: 10.1109/NC.2017.8263269.

Papageorgiou, A., Strigkos, M., Politou, E., Alepis, E., Solanas, A., Patsakis, C. (2018). Security and privacy analysis of mobile health applications: The alarming state of practice. *IEEE Access.*, 6, 9390–9403. DOI: 10.1109/ACCESS.2018.2799522.

Rejeb, A., Treiblmaier, H., Rejeb, K., Zailani, S. (2021). Blockchain research in healthcare: A bibliometric review and current research trends. *J. Data Inf. Manag.*, 3, 109–124. DOI: 10.1007/s42488-021-00046-2.

Romanou, A. (2018). The necessity of the implementation of privacy by design in sectors where data protection concerns arise. *Comput. Law Secur. Rev.*, 34, 99–110. DOI: 10.1016/j.clsr.2017.05.021.

Sharma, Y. and Balamurugan, B. (2020). Preserving the privacy of electronic health records using Blockchain. *Procedia Comput. Sci.*, 173, 171–180. DOI: 10.1016/j.procs.2020.06.021.

Sharma, K., Singh, H., Sharma, D.K., Kumar, A., Nayyar, A., Krishnamurthi, R. (2021). Dynamic models and control techniques for drone delivery of medications and other healthcare items in COVID-19 hotspots. DOI: 10.1007/978-3-030-60039-6_1.

Shu, I.N. and Jahankhani, H. (2017). The impact of the new european general data protection regulation (GDPR) on the information governance toolkit in health and social care with special reference to primary care in England. *2017 Cybersecurity and Cyberforensics Conference (CCC)*, 31–37. DOI: 10.1109/CCC.2017.16.

Singh, H., Talapula, D.K., Alind. (2019). IoT based real time road traffic monitoring and tracking system for hilly regions. *Int. J. Eng. Adv. Technol.*, 8(5), 2199–2205.

Sun, Z., Wang, Y., Shu, M., Liu, R., Zhao, H. (2019). Differential privacy for data and model publishing of medical data. *IEEE Access.*, 7, 152103–152114. DOI: 10.1109/ACCESS.2019.2947295.

Tian, H., He, J., Ding, Y. (2019). Medical data management on Blockchain with privacy. *J. Med. Syst.*, 43. DOI: 10.1007/s10916-018-1144-x.

Ul Hassan, M., Rehmani, M.H., Chen, J. (2020). Differential privacy in Blockchain technology: A futuristic approach. *J. Parallel Distrib. Comput.*, 145, 50–74. DOI: 10.1016/j.jpdc.2020.06.003.

Usman, M. and Qamar, U. (2020). Secure electronic medical records storage and sharing using Blockchain technology. *Procedia Comput. Sci.*, 174, 321–327. DOI: 10.1016/j.procs.2020.06.093.

Wahlstrom, K., Ulhaq, A., Burmeister, O. (2020). Privacy by design: A holochain exploration. *Australas. J. Inf. Syst.*, 24, 1–9. DOI: 10.3127/AJIS.V24I0.2801.

Yue, X., Wang, H., Jin, D., Li, M., Jiang, W. (2016). Healthcare data gateways: Found healthcare intelligence on Blockchain with novel privacy risk control. *J. Med. Syst.*, 40. DOI: 10.1007/s10916-016-0574-6.

Zhang, A. and Lin, X. (2018). Towards secure and privacy-preserving data sharing in e-health systems via consortium Blockchain. *J. Med. Syst.*, 42. DOI: 10.1007/s10916-018-0995-5.

8

Decentralized Smart Healthcare Systems Using Blockchain and AI

Patients, developers, vendors and legislators all face substantial challenges as a result of increased data availability and rapid innovations of intelligent machines in healthcare. Simple face photographs or videos are being transformed into effective records for predictive modeling, transforming whatever statistics that are more about people into medical sciences, courtesy of a unique, deep mastering or transferable learning algorithms. Patients now have little control over who has access to their medical records and are ignorant of the overall cost of the data they possess. Such revolutionary Blockchain generations will get society further to the idea that each patient record will be able to communicate changes to an open-source, community-wide relied-on ledger that is available and understood across enterprises with guaranteed integrity. This paper describes a Blockchain-enabled fragmented personal fitness facts ecosystem that enables unique drug discovery, biomarker development and preventative healthcare procedures, as well as secured personal records using Blockchain and deep learning technologies to connect users and providers of personal records with medical records.

8.1. Introduction to the healthcare system

Hospitals, dispensaries and primary healthcare departments are all distinct environments in which to work. Healthcare is complex, and people must be knowledgeable about a wide range of topics, including hospital forms, patient care, benefits, healthcare providers and legal difficulties. This guide will help people learn essential healthcare ideas so they may improve employee performance and understand the system.

For a color version of all figures in this chapter, see www.iste.co.uk/choudhury/blockchain.zip.

Chapter written by R.S.M. Lakshmi PATIBANDLA, Arepalli Peda GOPI, V. Lakshman NARAYANA and B. Tarakeswara RAO.

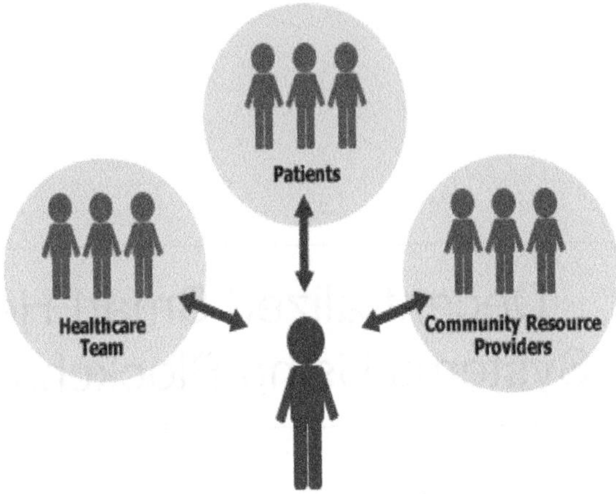

Figure 8.1. *Healthcare system relationships*

To be effective at work, people are well aware of the healthcare system. Users can collaborate in a variety of groupings, as seen in the diagram below. When people engage mostly with health professionals, users have to appreciate medical centers, possible treatments, as well as the roles of each team. People who work with patients must now be familiar with different types of insurance, how to assist uninsured people and how to protect patient privacy and rights. People will need to know what resources are available in their communities and how to get in touch with them.

8.1.1. *Introduction to AI*

Expert systems have also lately made headlines in the medical field, creating a heated discussion about whether AI doctors will ever be able to replace human doctors. Computers will not replace human doctors immediately, but AI will surely help physicians create good clinical decisions and may replace human judgment in some areas of healthcare (e.g. radiology). Recent successful AI applications in healthcare were made possible by the increased availability of healthcare data or the massive development in advanced analytics algorithms. Effective AI tools can extract clinically significant knowledge contained in vast amounts of data, assisting clinical decision-making (Al-Megren et al. 2018; Grishin et al. 2019; Han et al. 2019; Alsalamah and Nuzzolese 2020; Efremova and Teichmann 2020). The advantages of AI have been extensively studied in the scholarly literature. AI can use effective methods that can "learn" features from a big amount of healthcare data and then apply the results to improve modern medicine. It may also be able to learn from feedback and self-correct to enhance accuracy. Intelligent machines may support physicians by providing up-to-date medical information in the form of articles, textbooks and clinical procedures, allowing them to deliver proper patient care. Furthermore, any intelligence device could help with the decrease of diagnostic and treatment errors, is essential within human medicine. Furthermore, an AI device gathers useful data from a large number of patients to aid in creating real-time inferences for health risk alerts and predictions.

8.1.1.1. *Healthcare data*

To understand analogous people, connections among patient traits, with intended results, AI systems must be "trained" using data provided by clinical operations, such as screening, diagnosis or treatment assignment. Demographics, medical reports, electronic recordings from medical instruments, physical examinations, clinical laboratory tests and photos, along with many other things, are all samples of medical data (Alsalamah and Nuzzolese 2020).

8.1.2. *Introduction to Blockchain*

"Blockchains are tamper evident and tamper-resistant digital ledgers applied in a distributed manner (i.e. without a central repository) and normally without the central authority," according to the National Institute of Standards and Technology (NIST) ([e.g.] a bank, company or government). This enables any number of participants to store transactions in something like a smart contract within a team at its most basic level. A few transactions may be changed until they have been published when the Blockchain network is in normal operation. Although there are important distinctions, the terms Blockchain and distributed ledger technology (DLT) are frequently interchanged, especially when it comes to determining the solutions' business worth. A chain of data or transactions was defined as a group of situationally chained crypto signatures, which are related to from a hash, or preserved on shared ledgers, helped by a range of interconnected processes known as nodes. Nodes keep a copy of the entire chain on their computers, which is updated and maintained regularly.

Traditional programming, networks, databases and online applications are all built on well-known and proven underlying technologies including networking, hashing and encryption. It will approach architecture, trends, data exchange and implementation from a distinct angle. While Blockchain in healthcare is still in its infancy, early solutions have demonstrated the promise to lower healthcare costs, speed up business processes and increase knowledge access across disparate and diverse stakeholders working towards the same goal.

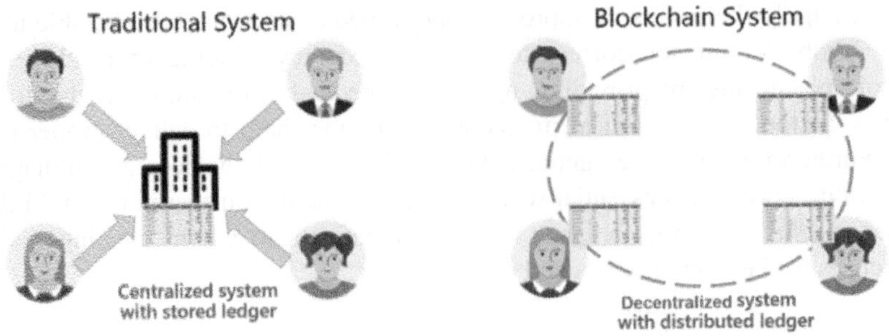

Figure 8.2. *Centralized system and decentralized Blockchain system*

No central authority has control over the content added to the Blockchain, which is a key characteristic of the technology. Rather, employing several consensual algorithms, the autonomous additions were chosen in such a peer-to-peer network. An extra key property of Blockchain is persistence. It is not viable to erase access when they have been approved into the Blockchain because it is distributed across multiple ledgers and processed by multiple repositories (Salah et al. 2019). Furthermore, several Blockchain technologies include the option of anonymity (or anonymization) as a desirable feature.

Concerning all recent and former chunks and using the author's hashing, Blockchain enables auditing and traceability. This results in a sequence of the block. The connections in the block were arranged into a Merkle tree (Chen et al. 2018), with every leaf's significance being confirmed against the notorious origin. The decision hierarchy may ensure its information's security just by placing the roots of a graph on this Blockchain.

8.2. Use of AI in healthcare systems

EHRs have supported the healthcare industry's digitalization, but the process has resulted in a plethora of challenges, including cognitive fatigue, repetitive paperwork and user burnout. Artificial intelligence has been used by EHR developers to create interfaces that are more intuitive and automate some of the repetitive tasks that previously took up a lot of a user's time. According to Adam Landman, MD, Vice President and Chief Information Officer of Brigham Healthcare, customers spend a significant amount of time on three things: clinical analysis, bar coding and scanning through the in-basket (Azaria et al. 2016; Destefanis et al. 2018; Kiktenko et al. 2018; Maxmen 2018; Tikhomirov et al. 2018). Natural language processing (NLP) approaches are insufficient; even though voice search and transcription could assist and enhance medical reporting. "We should be even more creative and consider adjustments like video recording a clinical session, similar to how police officers wear body cameras," claimed the data scientist. "After that, you can use artificial intelligence to catalog these recordings for possible information retrieval." Inside this future, software systems containing smart sensors will be brought to the bedside for doctors to use when placing orders, similar to using Siri, as well as Alexa at home.

Artificial intelligence could even manage routine tasks from its inbox, like narcotic prescriptions upon result updates. It can also help users complete their to-do lists by stressing items that require the clinician's attention, according to Landman. Healthcare executives are dealing with a plethora of hitherto unseen sales, cost and quality challenges. Artificial intelligence, they believe, is the key to better decision-making since it can provide faster observations or lower mistake tolerances.

These efforts could include augmented intelligence, which goes beyond artificial intelligence by allowing humans to make the most informed decision possible, even if they occasionally fail.

As a result, a growing number of business and analytics professionals are striving to incorporate artificial intelligence (AI) into their forecasting processes to better address these pressing concerns. These efforts have far too often failed spectacularly. Leaders have struggled to leverage analytics into current systems, integrate or change workflows, and convey the benefits of AI.

The first version of Medical Catalyst's Healthcare was primarily focused on its use cases that involve step as well as service prediction models. However, when used without expert guidance (self-service), the aforementioned methodology was nearly always inefficient, and its range was too limited, limiting its usefulness in healthcare (Medicine Catalyst's new healthcare service) (Yaji et al. 2018; Salah et al. 2019; Mattos et al. 2020). The AI provides a positive, disruptive product range or destinations to visit to address a broader range of market concerns (healthcare). Intelligence substantially broadens its diversity for application, but is used in situations in the workplace.

8.3. Use of Blockchain in healthcare systems

Blockchain networks may help with data privacy, diversity and transaction cost reduction. They can also help with the exactness of medication, bettering patient care with results, as well as integrating cross-border health records. This may be advantageous in an emergency since the hospital can contact data right away rather than having to acquire individual patient information (Woods 2018; Kumar Singh et al. 2020).

Blockchain networks can offer real-time medical supervision or knowledge upgrades by integrating these capabilities, while employing machine learning to evaluate sensor nodes (IoT). When linked to a database, it can be used by medical care providers, as well as a range of enterprises. As a result, healthcare workers now have easy access to patient records, which saves money and improves collaboration between hospitals.

Blockchains could still benefit the Health Information Exchange (HIE), as well as the Integrated for Health Care Enterprise. Integrating the system via functions such as insurance providers, financial and operating services, revenue cycles and suppliers could still significantly reduce back-office input data and maintenance expenses (Karafiloski and Mishev 2017; Kumar Singh et al. 2020). Additional benefits include data accuracy and security. Based on continual statistical pooling, localities will probably develop unified healthcare systems. Several benefits of expanding the healthcare system could eventually result in a reduction; there is a set of cases and online healthcare systems. Finally, Blockchain technology has the potential to be employed in a variety of data-driven healthcare sectors, including health records, claims, interoperability, patient access and supply chains.

8.4. History of medical care

A patient's medical history can be compiled using Blockchains. This longitudinal data can be maintained in blocks, providing useful information not only about individual patients, but also for other population segments. A distributed network aids care coordination between multiple service providers. For example, in a hypothetical situation, to get a patient's medical history, a physician may scan their smart wrists. That is especially significant in medical settings because the patient's information is sent in real time to the hospital and doctor, who then use the chain to gain access to healthcare accounts, including the data entered by the attending technician. Wearable devices rely on the IoT, which provides hospital-based diagnosis and treatment from anywhere. Furthermore, merging health data from mobile apps with genomes can provide useful information about subpopulations that are vulnerable to certain diseases or respond to specific medications.

8.4.1. *Health claims*

Another field that could benefit from modular design is health claims and insurance. Such are approved swiftly when connected to a Blockchain, saving time and money. Because patients' bank and healthcare bank deposits will be interconnected through the usage of Blockchain, data exchange methods, as well as networking devices could enable the fast settlement of disputes.

8.4.2. *Interoperability*

Medical records have traditionally been disconnected and stored in service provider silos. This is due to fact that electronic health records (EHRs) were designed episode by episode, without taking into consideration the linkages needed for lifetime records or many service providers, and hence lack linkages, common designs and standards. There is no system in place for sharing medical data with stakeholders or even patients. As a result, the patient's regular proven records cannot be modified into such at other periods if competing health services remain accessible. Both patients and medical care providers benefit greatly from interoperability. Population health projects are made possible by data interoperability, as to help with these large-scale initiatives, a chain may also be used to collect massive volumes of health information.

8.4.3. *Exposure to healthcare*

Patients have access to their medical records, which is another advantage of a data collection agreement. This is reliant on the portability of healthcare data, which can be achieved if regulatory and legal standards have been completed. Hospitals offer their most push medicines if a medical Blockchain technology has been related to more relevant clinical studies. Patients will be better informed and able to discuss the best treatment options with medical doctors based on research rather than traditional knowledge. A decentralized system is used for medical data integration by providing safe yet secure medical data facts, synchronizing records and granting patient access while checking user compliance.

8.4.4. *Supply chains*

Blockchains are also used to connect patients, network operators or enterprises across supply chains in order to track or fulfill requests in real time. Consumers should educate themselves on the efficacy, origins and adverse effects of the ingredients in their prescriptions. As a result, supply chain efficiency and quality control may improve. A manufacturing process called Blockchain can track products back to the manufacturer, and manage vendor or customer payments, lowering costs and eliminating human error. Blockchain provides numerous potential in the healthcare area. It may lead to integrated healthcare data, which will help governments establish national healthcare systems. For healthcare, Blockchains can virtually likely be put to a wide range of applications. The Blockchain, we believe, will have the same impact on the medical system that the Internet did on the media.

8.5. Literature review

In the realm of healthcare, there are currently no AI models accessible. Artificial intelligence has made lives better for patients, clinicians and healthcare executives by performing tasks that were previously performed by people at a fraction of the cost. AI has a variety of uses in the medical industry. The healthcare system in the United States is in serious need of an overhaul. From chronic diseases and cancer to radiography and quality assurance, there is an almost limitless opportunity to use technology to deliver increasingly precise, efficient and impactful treatments at precisely the correct time during a client's treatment. Artificial intelligence is positioned to be the spark that enables changes throughout the whole system as payment methods grow, clients demand more out of healthcare providers or the availability of data continues to rise.

Diagnostic decision-making with analytics systems has a variety of disadvantages compared to AI. When learning algorithms communicate with one another, they can become more exact and accurate, giving humans unique insights into diagnosis, treatment variations and patient outcomes. Leading academics and clinical instructors discussed the 12 innovations, as well as other aspects of the healthcare sector; another, very certainly to see even a significant impact from machine learning throughout the next quarter of a century in the same week, the 2018 World Medical Innovation Forum (WMIF) on machine learning took place, and was featured by Members Healthcare.

Although EHRs have benefited the healthcare industry's digitization efforts, the change has resulted in a plethora of problems, including cognitive fatigue, endless paperwork and user burnout. Healthcare architects are already employing artificial intelligence to produce more user-friendly interfaces and automate some time-consuming repetitive tasks. Clinical reporting, patient registration and sifting among both the in/out seem to be three activities that certain individuals expend significant amounts of time on.

NLP techniques are insufficient for clinical documentation, despite the reality that speech recognition or synthesis can aid it. Following on from his advocation for the use of video cameras in clinical encounters, Landman continued: "Users can then categorize similar recordings using AI and machine learning for possible information retrieval. In the future, virtual assistants to medics would be brought to a hospital, similarly to how we use Siri and Alexa at home, and will be able to submit orders using embedded intelligence." Artificial intelligence could then handle everyday demands from the inbox, such as diabetic supplies following result updates. It can also assist users in completing their to-do lists by stressing items that require immediate attention from the doctor.

Antibiotic resistance is becoming a growing issue for people all over the world, even though the excessive use of these life-saving treatments stimulates the creation of antibiotic-resistant superbugs. Multidrug-resistant bacteria may wreak havoc in hospitals, killing thousands of people every year. The United States health service spends $5 billion each year and puts the lives of over 30,000 individuals in jeopardy. Data from electronic health records could help detect infection patterns and identify people who are at risk, before they display symptoms. The use of machine learning and artificial intelligence to drive these analytics will improve their accuracy and provide health firms with easier, more accurate notifications.

"Artificial Intelligence technologies will meet contagion and be in command of antibiotic conflict expectations," says Erica Shenoy, MD, Ph.D., and Associate Chief of the MGH Infection Control Unit. "If they don't, we're doomed." It would be a tragedy if hospitals sat on mounds of EHR data and did not do anything with it, if the industry did not develop better, faster clinical trial design, and if EHRs did not use the data they generate.

Making pathologic vision analysis even more precise, "An EHR's pathology outcome accounts for 70–75 percent of the data. The more specific we can be, and the sooner we can reach an accurate diagnosis, the better. That's something AI and digital pathology can help with." Suppliers may be able to spot things that would otherwise be missed, mostly by sensory systems through procedures that can dig deeper into an input image on incredibly huge digital photographs. "We would finally at a point where we can predict whether cancer will advance quickly or slowly, and how that can affect how patients are treated using an algorithm rather than clinical staging or histopathology grade," Golden said. "That would be a huge step forward." According to humans, artificial intelligence will increase efficiency by detecting features of interest on slides before a human doctor evaluating the material. "AI will scan through presentations and point us to the important information so we can figure out what's important and what's not," the researcher explains. This reduces pathologist costs, while increasing the value of the time they spend on each patient.

8.6. Bringing intelligence to medical devices and machines

Smart devices are sweeping the consumer sector, from real-time imagery from within refrigerators through autos, which can identify whether drivers are focused.

Smart devices are important in the medical business for tracking patients in the ICU and elsewhere. Artificial intelligence may improve the ability to predict deterioration, detect the imminent development of sepsis or identify the onset of complications, resulting in lower costs associated with hospital-acquired diseases. "We're talking about aggregating fragmented data from throughout the healthcare system, merging it, and producing simply one warning that prompts an ICU doctor to intervene early on," noted Mark Michalski, MD, Executive Director of the MGH & BWH Centre for Clinical Data Science. Integrating intelligent systems into specific gadgets may make professionals' perceptions easier, and patients can receive treatment as quickly as feasible.

In monitoring systems, wearable tech, or portable tools, almost every consumer will soon have access to a device equipped with sensors capable of recording pertinent health data. When people are outside, they generate additional healthcare data, from cell phones with step trackers to wearables that can detect pulses all over the world. Researchers may be able to gain a unique perspective on health promotion by analyzing results, as well as merging this with the information provided from individuals using an app or other personal monitoring equipment. Artificial intelligence (AI) can assist in the extraction of important facts from such a large and varied data source. Persuading patients to share statistics from such close, ongoing monitoring, according to Omar Arnaout, MD, Co-Director of such a Cognitive Neurology Health Center, but an associate surgeon of BWH, may require some extra effort.

"We've been quite progressive as a nation without this electronic data." People may become more cautious about who to cooperate with when firms such as Cambridge Analytica, as well as Facebook, grow. Patients, on the other hand, are more inclined to trust their doctors than a global corporation such as Facebook, according to him, which could help to relieve any concerns about providing data to large-scale research projects. According to Arnaout, as our treatments are often temporal, and the records that customers get are so imprecise, there was a decent chance (personal statistics) have a major impact. "Collecting granular data frequently enhances the likelihood that the data will help us provide better patient care."

Experts agree that photos taken with mobile phones and other consumer-grade devices would be a fantastic supplement to clinical quality imaging, especially for underprivileged populations in developing nations. This is part of leveraging the power of portable technology, according to experts. Every year, camera phones improve in resolution, and they can now produce photographs that artificial intelligence algorithms may evaluate. The first specialties to benefit from this innovation were dermatology and ophthalmology.

Researchers in the United Kingdom have also developed a system that analyzes linguistic renderings in addition to identifying brain illnesses. The method can detect distinct features such as a child's jawline, eye and nose alignment, and other characteristics that may suggest a craniofacial aberration. This software is presently capable of matching common pictures to over 90 diseases, allowing clinicians to make better selections. "Most people have pocket-sized, powerful gadgets with a variety of sensors built-in," HadiShafiee, Ph.D., director of BWH's Laboratory of Micro/Nanomedicine and Digital Health, said.

> This is an once-in-a-lifetime chance for us. Almost every major industry player has started to integrate artificial intelligence (AI) software and technology into their services. This is not a coincidence. In this virtual era, researchers acquire over 2.5 million gigabytes of data every day. People will be able to give even more convenient, faster, smarter solutions by mixing this technology with AI, according to mobile phone manufacturers.

8.7. Using artificial intelligence to transform clinical decision-making in hospitals

In the same way that the healthcare business is moving away from fee-for-service, reactive treatment is being phased out. Every good feeling connected with avoiding chronic diseases, costly acute events and unanticipated deterioration, as well as reimbursement systems, are eventually assisting in the development of mechanisms that will allow proactive, predictive therapies.

Predictive modeling or medical data-gathering systems that alert clinicians to difficulties well before they would otherwise note some need to intervene will be supported by artificial intelligence, which may offer the majority of the basis for such a progress.

AI will also provide early indications of disorders along with seizures, as sepsis usually needs extensive analysis of large datasets. According to Brandon Westover, MD, Ph.D., Director of the MGH Clinical Data Animation Centre, computer experience has aided clinicians in determining whether to continue caring for patients who have recently entered a coma after cardiac arrest. Typically, clinicians must visually evaluate EEG data from such people, according to the study. The procedure takes time and is subjective, with different outcomes depending on the clinician's competence and experience.

"Trends may have been emerging in these patients," he speculated. "When we're waiting to see if others have healed, humans take data for 10 minutes of tracking.

Trying to figure out if it's better than ten seconds of data collected 24 hours ago is like trying to tell if your hair is becoming longer. However, if you have an AI system and a lot of data from a lot of patients, it's a lot easier to correlate what you're seeing to long-term trends and maybe identify little changes that can influence your treatment decisions."

Among the key areas of use of AI in data analysis are clinical treatment, risk assessment and advanced alarms. Automation must facilitate the birth of a global era of studied groups and fascinating scientific advances via medical services, while enhancing a generation of innovative products. Furthermore, systems can make physicians more conscious of subtleties, more impactful when distributing care and thus more intent to get ahead of imminent trends, all while inspiring a generation of innovations or components that make clinicians more aware of complexities, more successful in delivering treatments and thus even more capable of staying ahead of current threats.

8.7.1. *Advantages of Blockchain in healthcare systems*

Blockchain is a game-changing commercial information-transfer system that has swept the globe, especially in the financial sector. Its huge success inside a range of organizations has caused alarm in the healthcare field. The "current tool that will handle healthcare's impending issues" is being referred to as an "action plan towards compatibility", but if the mystery continues, it will take much longer. Blockchain, on the other hand, does have the potential to make a huge difference in the delivery of universal healthcare. Satoshi Nakamoto, a pseudonymous individual (or group), invented Blockchain in 2008 as a major component of the digital currency bitcoin.

With the technical language out of the way, Blockchain is simply a peer-to-peer system to exchange records, and archives all image retrieval in numerical order. It preserves records in the form of transfers or exchanges that may be transmitted and traded between authorized individuals who can add to it as needed. Is it not self-explanatory? However, here is where Blockchain stands out: these authorized people are unable to delete or edit any records, and no transfer may be accomplished until they have confirmed it.

Blockchain is a three-part peer-to-peer distributed ledger technology:

1) Decentralized peer-to-peer framework: in such a decentralized model, nodes created by network members store an identical copy of the Blockchain and can validate and certify digital transactions for the network.

2) Shared ledger: all electronic transfers are recorded in a shared ledger by network participants. They run algorithms that verify the proposed transaction, which is then added to the shared ledger until a majority of citizens approve it.

3) Digital transaction: the layers, which can be processed on a Blockchain, are data or a mobile platform. Each transaction is grouped into a "block", which includes a cryptographic hash that allows for the sequential insertion of transactions. In most cases of AI in healthcare, sensitive data is dispersed across multiple networks, and it may not be available when it is most required. Because of its order to maintain information sharing, it has been advised that current health services be altered.

Blockchain has already gone through its "modernization phase" and is currently at the "height of magnified prospect", as per the newest Gartner Hype Cycle, because it has the potential to transform how we think about healthcare and data. One of the most essential advantages of Blockchain in healthcare is the lack of a fixed network, in our opinion. A database is always made up of bits and bytes. If the database's contents are saved in just a network's hard disk, everyone who sees it can corrupt the data.

Blockchain technology will not require a central administrator since sophisticated cryptography will eliminate the necessity for one. In addition, all customers have complete control over their personal information and transactions. Blockchain can help simplify medical records and enable safe sharing, despite healthcare working with sensitive patient data that requires quick access to information. Blockchain enables access control, scalability or data protection in one fell stroke. Although the concept of Blockchain in healthcare is innovative, it will not be a panacea for data management issues.

Instead, Blockchain would have been introduced in such a systematic fashion. Blockchain is also on the to-do list of only 5% of CIOs and 12% of industry leaders. Hence, despite the hoopla, we must educate ourselves on Blockchain's actual applicability in healthcare:

1) Medical data on a single patient, which is retained for the rest of their life

Longitudinal patient records, such as inpatient, ambulatory or wearable data, could be established using Blockchain, allowing physicians to better deliver care by aggregating episodes, sickness registries, lab tests and treatments.

2) Participant master indices

It is usual that health data should never be misaligned nor duplicated. Furthermore, each EHR has a distinct schema for each region, leading to a wide range of methods for inputting and modifying even the most basic data sets. The complete data collection was encoded to either a Blockchain or a bitcoin on the Blockchain, except the username and password. The user should look for the address; there could be multiple addresses and keys, but they will all lead to the same patient identification.

3) The evaluation of claims

Because Blockchain was built on validation, the claims could be continuously analyzed, and the network can judge how a contract is carried out. There will be simple designs or forgeries, although there will not be a requirement at the time.

4) Managing the supply chain

Health systems may use Blockchain-based contracts to track inventory phases throughout their full life-cycle, including how the transaction is progressing, whether the contract is functional, and whether any delays have occurred.

5) Interoperability

The promise of Blockchain, interoperability, may be fulfilled by cognition APIs to protect EHR interoperability and data storage. When the Blockchain network is accessible with authorized suppliers outside in a secured and systematic way, the complications and the duty of recovering data are eliminated.

Apart from these applications, Blockchain technology has the potential to improve sales cycle management, medicine supply management, clinical trials and fraud prevention. Each of the Blockchain's capabilities in healthcare is largely determined by how eager healthcare providers are to invest in the appropriate technology infrastructure. The cost of Blockchain is considerable; there are doubts about how it will interact using current technology, but there is a lot of discussion about its cultural adoption. However, one thing is certain: so far this year, Blockchain has taken the global healthcare business by storm, and there have been significant Blockchain investments. With so many possibilities, it is no surprise that Blockchain is poised to become one of the largest essential foundations throughout the virtual environment. Who knows, it may even transform the big data landscape in the future.

8.8. Results of existing models

The medical industry will be able to provide better quality treatment, lower prices and modernize healthcare by integrating its state of the art inside these technologies. AI requires data, and Blockchain enables the storage of encrypted data. All reasoning involved inside this computational decision-making phase will be determined using Blockchain technology. The "near future" holds the promise of a general agreement on allegations, data protection transition and knowing the next models from the provider–payer perspective. In addition to the required secrecy, according to TejAnand of the University Of Texas McCombs School Of Business, Blockchain can help in healthcare by removing needless jobs, rework and reconciliation. If AI was employed in a predicted healthcare setting, users could control operations to reach the correct quality of service intensity. The information would be shared with the appropriate person – a clinician, a patient or a caregiver – in the most efficient manner possible. Blockchain is vital towards Covid-safe medical care. The integration of Blockchain and AI capabilities makes it easier to better diagnose and treat Covid-19 patients, as well as develop clinical guidelines based on pandemic objectives.

Blockchain networks can be used to share data from clinical labs, hospitals, primary care providers, physicians and other sources, while maintaining privacy and security. Data will be analyzed using artificial intelligence (AI) solutions. This concept is effective for risk management, and also boosts research and development of novel medications.

8.9. Conclusion

In the years to come, Blockchain and AI technologies will accelerate and transform the sector. Other tech behemoths, such as Apple, Amazon and Google, are foraying into the healthcare sector. In conclusion, the healthcare industry is rapidly increasing, and the consequences will be seen shortly.

8.10. References

Al-Megren, S., Alsalamah, S., Altoaimy, L., Alsalamah, H., Soltanisehat, L. (2018). Blockchain use cases in digital sectors: A review of the literature. *2018 IEEE International Conference on Internet of Things (iThings) and IEEE Green Computing and Communications (GreenCom) and IEEE Cyber, Physical and Social Computing (CPSCom) and IEEE Smart Data (SmartData)*, 1417–1424. doi:10.1109/cybermatics2018.2018.00242.

Alsalamah, S. and Nuzzolese, E. (2020). Promising Blockchain technology applications and use case designs for the identification of multinational victims of mass disasters. *Frontiers in Blockchain*, 3, 34. doi:10.3389/fbloc.2020.00034.

Azaria, A., Ekblaw, A., Vieira, T., Lippman, A. (2016). Medrec: Using Blockchain for medical data access and permission management. *2016 2nd International Conference on Open and Big Data (OBD)*, 25–30.

Chen, J., Ma, X., Du, M., Wang, Z. (2018). A Blockchain application for medical information sharing. *2018 IEEE International Symposium on Innovation and Entrepreneurship (TEMS-ISIE)*, 1–7.

Destefanis, G., Marchesi, M., Ortu, M., Tonelli, R., Bracciali, A., Hierons, R. (2018). Smart contracts vulnerabilities: A call for Blockchain software engineering? *Proc. Int. Workshop Blockchain Oriented Softw. Eng. (IWBOSE)*, 19–25.

Efremova, M. and Teichmann, S.A. (2020). Computational methods for single-cell omics across modalities. *Nat. Methods*, 17, 14–17. doi: 10.1038/s41592-019-0692-4.

Grishin, D., Obbad, K., Church, G.M. (2019). Data privacy in the age of personal genomics. *Nat. Biotechnol.*, 37, 1115–1117. doi: 10.1038/s41587-019-0271-3.

Han, X., Wang, Y., Wei, J., Han, W. (2019). Multi-antigen-targeted chimeric antigen receptor T cells for cancer therapy. *J. Hematol. Oncol.*, 12, 128. doi: 10.1186/s13045-019-0813-7.

Karafiloski, E. and Mishev, A. (2017). Blockchain solutions for big data challenges: A literature review. *Proceedings of the IEEE EUROCON 2017 – 17th International Conference on Smart Technologies*, Piscataway, NJ, 763–768.

Kiktenko, E.O., Pozhar, N.O., Anufriev, M.N., Trushechkin, A.S., Yunusov, R.R., Kurochkin, Y.V., Lvovsky, A.I., Fedorov, A.K. (2018). Quantum-secured blockchain. *Quantum Sci. Technol.*, 3(3), 035004. doi: 10.1088/2058-9565/aabc6b.

Kumar Singh, S., Rathore, S., Park, J.H. (2020). Block IoT intelligence: A Blockchain-enabled intelligent IoT architecture with artificial intelligence. *Future Generation Comput. Syst.*, 110, 721–743. doi: 10.1016/j.future.2019.09.002.

Mattos, D.M.F., Krief, F., Rueda, S.J. (2020). Blockchain and artificial intelligence for network security. *Ann. Telecommun.*, 75, 101–102. doi: 10.1007/s12243-020-00754-7.

Maxmen, A. (2018). AI researchers embrace bitcoin technology to share medical data. *Nature* [Online]. Available at: www.nature.com/articles/d41586-018-02641-7.

Salah, K., Rehman, M.H.U., Nizamuddin, N., Al-Fuqaha, A. (2019). Blockchain for AI: Review and open research challenges. *IEEE Access*, 7, 10127–10149. doi: 10.1109/ACCESS.2018.2890507.

Sharath, Y., Kajal, B., Neelima, B. (2018). Privacy preserving in Blockchain based on partial homomorphic encryption system for AI applications. *2018 IEEE 25th International Conference on High Performance Computing Workshop (HIPCW)*, 81–85.

Tikhomirov, S., Voskresenskaya, E., Ivanitskiy, I., Takhaviev, R., Marchenko, E., Alexandrov, Y. (2018). Smartcheck: Static analysis of ethereum smart contracts. *Proc. IEEE/ACM 1st Int. Workshop Emerg. Trends Softw. Eng. Blockchain (WETSEB)*, May/June, 9–16.

Woods, J. (2018) Blockchain: Rebalancing & amplifying the power of AI and machine learning (ML) [Online]. Available at: http://medium.com/crypto-oracle/blockchain-rebalancing-amplifying-the power-of-ai-and-machine-learning-mlaf95616e9ad9.

9

Component-based Healthcare Software Application Using Blockchain

Software technology plays an important role in our lifestyles. This technology affects our activities in many areas such as education, the car industry, administration, games, healthcare, etc. The primary aim of the software industry is to produce a high-quality and low-cost software system in good time. To achieve this goal, many software companies follow the component-based software engineering approach to develop software rather than traditional approaches. The component-based approach is an emerging technology for software development. Its main aim is to develop a software system by selecting the appropriate software components from a repository as per the requirement specification and assemble all of the components with a well-defined software architecture. Healthcare software systems are gaining attention from software developers as they are being increasingly used in day-to-day life. In the present scenario, monitoring our health has become a part of many people's lifestyles. This means that customers need to search for reliable and secure healthcare software. The main challenges of health applications are to manage data safety. Hence, we need a technology that provides confidentially and security for healthcare information. Blockchain is one of the technologies that can be used to secure our data and increase our trust in the application. Further, it is becoming popular because of its features, which include security, decentralization, immutability and transparency. Many healthcare standards such as life-cycle models and design methodologies give the best software practices and design principles to secure our application. In this chapter, we discuss the life-cycles of software development through the component-based software engineering approach. Further, we discuss how to create a Blockchain-based repository that stores software component and also discuss how Blockchain technology helps to secure our data in healthcare applications. The proposed software development life-cycle model ensures the security of user data and also improves the quality of healthcare applications.

For a color version of all figures in this chapter, see www.iste.co.uk/choudhury/blockchain.zip.

Chapter written by Nisha PAL and Dharmendra Kumar YADAV.

9.1. Introduction

Today, software is being used everywhere, such as in the education, health, transportation, banking, sports and communication sectors etc. Software is required to operate computers, airplanes, mobiles, TVs, cars and even children's toys. It has a great impact on our daily lives and society. It supports comfortable living, along with monitoring facilities. In recent years, the healthcare sector has grown rapidly and has started to use software technology. Software technology has ensured that digitalized records are more effectively accessible when needed. The appropriate use of medical software will prove to be a boon for the health industry. It provides better accessibility for patient records, easy collaboration between physicians and easy to track patient health records, which all contribute to the best treatment (Katuwal et al. 2018; Ullah et al. 2020). Therefore, the effect of these applications is to shorten the patient's treatment time, save money and effort, resolve the problem of unnecessary visits, and maintain and update the patient's medical history. However, implementing healthcare software faces various challenges, such as how to choose better software methodology, how to incorporate user requirements into the design, how to trust in the medical software, how to easily adopt changes in technologies and culture, and also how to fix security issues. Healthcare solutions provide different types of software services, such as electronic health record services, practice management software, hospital management systems, billing software, lab information management software, etc., and tries to fulfill patient needs. But all of these software services have not increased the trust and transparency between the patient and the physician.

Software engineering methodologies play an important role in building a large and complex healthcare application. Software engineering can be defined as the study of the software process, principles and methodology applied in any real scenario of software development (Lalband et al. 2019). It helps to reduce the complexity of large software development, minimize software cost, deliver on time, handle bugs, and fulfill user expectations and needs. A proper software model (known as a software development life-cycle model) plays a vital role in developing software. Effective software models in software engineering help to build, design, develop, test, maintain and evolve any software systematically. It is a framework that helps to pre-plan. The software industry that tells us how to create a software product. Software development life-cycle (SDLC) is a group of various phases that helps us to understand the process of building software. It helps the developer to understand project context and user requirements. Hence, the project's success always requires the best SDLC model according to its needs. An effective SDLC model provides a good software project within a certain timeframe, at lower cost, with less effort, without going over budget.

In the 1960s, there was no method or framework for the development of the software process model. The developer collects all of the information related to software in text form. Hence, it was not able to properly understand what exactly the user wanted. Due to this, developing software was time-consuming and needed more effort. But today, the definition of the software development process is different. They follow standards and methods to create any kind of project. SDLC uses these standards to collect and analyze requirements related to the development process systematically. There are various SDLC methodologies, such as the waterfall model, iterative model, prototyping model, spring model, agile model, etc., which are used for software development. Each SDLC model is different from the other. But these models are older and do not give more functionality to the user or support rapidly changing requirements. Today, due to more expectations of user requirements, the developer is bound to create large and complex software. These traditional models are not fit to develop large and complex software and never give better quality and accuracy. Hence, the developer needs to choose another advanced SDLC model technique that removes the above issues and uses less time, cost and effort to develop software. It also ensures that transparency between the developers is maintained, developing speed is enhanced and the risk factor is minimized. At the end, users get a high-quality product that fulfills user requirements. This advanced SDLC model technique is based on component-based software engineering (CBSE).

CBSE is an advance development approach in which software products are developed by selecting reliable and reusable components, and assembled using the appropriate software architecture (Mahmood et al. 2007; Vale et al. 2016). Here, the component is various software modules, packages, self-unit codes that are executed, verified and deployed independently. The main aim of adopting this technique is to increase productivity, lower cost and time to market, and improve performance and quality. This new concept is different from the traditional approach, where software is not developed from scratch. The CBSE approach consists of two life-cycles that work in parallel, one is a component-based development life-cycle and another is a system development life-cycle through component. When a developer wants to create any software using the CBSE approach, they search for the desired components in the software repository. If the desired components are present in the repository, then they assemble these components and construct a software product. If the desired component is not presented in the repository, then they create it from scratch. The development of an SDLC based on CBSE plays an important role in providing better-quality and cost-effective software (Aoyama 1998; Cai et al. 2000). A better development life-cycle model helps to reduce time, cost and effort and increases the performance and quality of the software. Although this approach increases the software's productivity and performance, it does not increase reliability and trust in them as the selection of expected software components to develop the software is not always trustworthy and reliable. Hence, the developer needs to improve our software development life-cycle with advance technologies such as Blockchain, cloud computing, artificial intelligence (AI) and Internet of Things (IoT) that increase the reliability and trust in them. Figure 9.1 shows the constructions of software development based on CBSE.

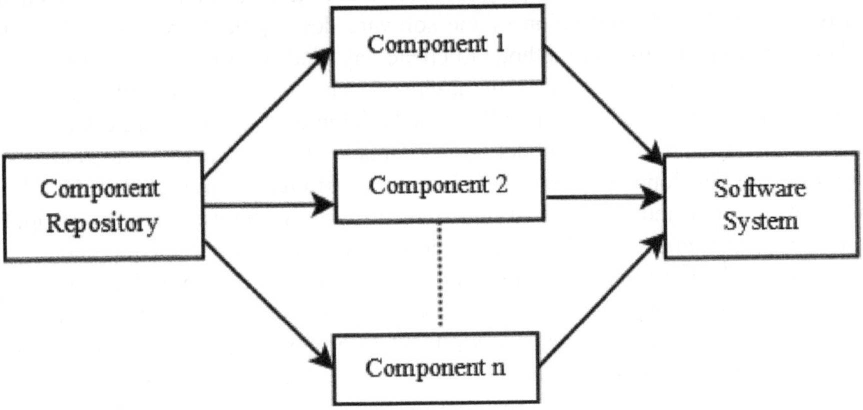

Figure 9.1. *Component-based software development (Cai et al. 2000)*

Many research organizations are trying to develop a software system with the latest technology to increase our trust and secure data exchanges. Blockchain technology is a system that has the above features. A Blockchain is defined as a distributed digital ledger. It contains several blocks. These blocks are interlinked by hash cryptography in a peer-to-peer network. Every block of the Blockchain contains a block number, time stamp, nonce, data in the form of Merkle root and hash of the previous block, as shown in Figure 9.2. Every block is immutable, so there is no possibility of malicious attacks in the future. This technology was firstly introduced by Haber and Stornetta in 1991, and the first application was introduced by Satoshi Nakamoto in 2008 in the form of cryptocurrency for peer-to-peer transactions, known as Bitcoin (Nakamoto 2009). In Blockchain, data can be stored as a block that contains any type of data such as text, video and any kind of transaction. When a new block wants to join this Blockchain, its information is broadcast over the entire peer network, where miners are ready to mine this new block. After mining, a valid block is added to the Blockchain. Each Blockchain contains a set of rules known as a consensus algorithm (PoW, PoS). With the help of a consensus algorithm, the miners validate the new block and decide which block is added to or discarded from the Blockchain. This technology is becoming more popular because of its features, which include security, decentralization, immutability and transparency. Blockchain has the potential to solve many problems related to healthcare applications, such as a lack of disability of transition, trust and security for the patient record. It increases the trust without any intermediaries and provides a new business model. Due to its potential, Blockchain technology has attracted the healthcare industry to develop a healthcare application using it. It can be used in different fields of healthcare such as supply chain management of medical goods, patient record management, pharmaceutical research, telemedicine, etc. (Katuwal et al. 2018; De Aguiar et al. 2020). In Blockchain technology, data is stored in immutable form and cannot be deleted or altered. Hence, using Blockchain technology in healthcare software increases the trust, reliability, traceability and security of the patient record.

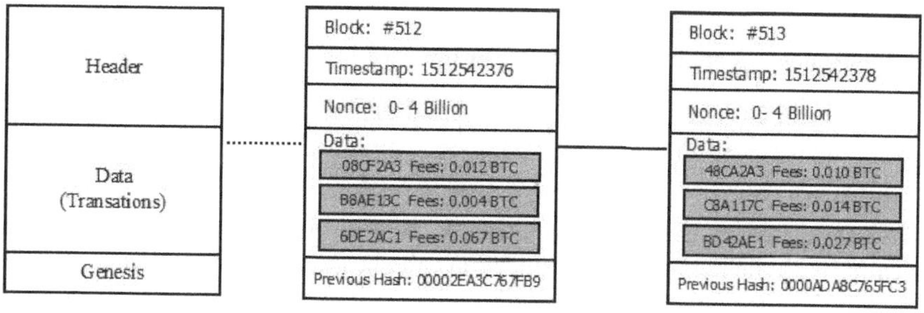

Figure 9.2. *Structure of Blockchain*

In recent years, the healthcare industry has started adopting new technology that increases the quality of care and fast recovery rate from the disease. Upcoming new technologies such as cloud computing, AI, Blockchain and IoT are being used in the medical field, which provide more benefits for developing healthcare applications. Healthcare IT solutions promise to improve interoperability between patient and doctor, reduce the overall cost of healthcare delivery and increase the accessibility of patient records according to their requirement. The main focus of this chapter is to identify the factor that affects healthcare quality. Many healthcare policies provide the best software practices and design principles to secure applications. When developing any healthcare software system, cost, time, effort, trust and security are the main factors that affect the development process. An effective SDLC helps to reduce these kinds of difficulties. SDLC is defined as a tool based on the project context and is helpful for producing high-quality software. A better life-cycle improves the quality of care for the patient. It decreases manpower hours, treatment costs and supports easy accesses to patient information in a timely manner. In this chapter, we have discussed the life-cycles of software development through the component-based software engineering approach. Further, we discuss how to create a Blockchain-based repository that stores software components in the form of blocks and discuss how Blockchain technology helps to secure the health-related data of a patient in healthcare applications and increase the trust in the patient record. The proposed component-based software development life-cycle with Blockchain ensures that our data is secured and also improves the quality of healthcare applications.

The rest of this chapter is organized as follows: section 9.2 provides a literature review. Section 9.3 explores the software development models in detail. Section 9.4 describes the proposed model using Blockchain technology. Section 9.5 presents a comparative study among different software development life-cycle models and section 9.6 concludes the proposed work and provides future research directions.

9.2. Literature review

Every new technology has helped to increase human productivity, performance and its prosperity. Many industries have been attracted due to this new technology, and the healthcare industry is one of them. Technology has brought about massive changes in the healthcare industry today. Due to this, users can now choose the best medical devices according to their requirement. The increases in demand for software related to healthcare applications provide many benefits to patients and doctors. With the help of these applications, the hospital can easily create a database related to the patient's medical records and treatment records; the doctors can easily study diseases and diagnose them quickly and accurately. Using healthcare software and its applications, we can easily perform various activities, such as blood testing, brain testing, body scanning, Covid-19 testing, etc. Remote consultation and different mobile apps have also led to improving patient care and giving better results for the patient. The main aim of implementing healthcare applications is to provide a lower cost, minimize error, improve patient experiences, easily update their records and also trust these sensitive patient records. However, technology innovation and the high expectations of the patient create new challenges for the medical organization, such as quality, privacy, security and trust of the patient data. Hence, the user searches for better-quality products and services.

Healthcare applications always demand the best technology, methodology and a software development model to resolve the above problem. A proper software development cycle model is essential for any software to become successful. An SDLC model is a software engineering process used to design, develop, test and deploy any software system. In other words, we can say that SDLC is considered as a framework that provides a sequence of activities for the system developer, as well as system designer. SDLC contains different phases that are essential for developing any software system, such as requirement analysis, design, coding and testing. Different SDLC models are suitable for specific projects that depend on some conditions such as which organization uses it, the stability of the requirement, the risk factor, budget and time duration of the project (Rastogi 2015; Gajalakshmi 2016). It gives perspective characteristics that provide suggestions of how to develop a software system.

Finding an appropriate SDLC model is a very challenging task. An efficient SDLC model aids in the improvement of software product quality while reducing cost and time. Kneuper (2017) discussed various software development life-cycle models and provided a detailed overview of these models' development. This paper describes how SDLC affects the rise of software processes. According to the author, an effective life-cycle model resolves the productivity and scalability problem in software development time. The author also discussed a new type of life-cycle model known as Kanban and Devops. This new life-cycle model helps to decrease the process time and improve the quality of the software process. Ragunath et al. (2010) presented various life-cycle models and gave the comparative analysis between them. According to the authors, incident management, change management and release management are the key issues of any SDLC models. To resolve these issues, the authors have proposed a hypothetical model called SDLC model 2010. This model is based on the three-dimensional model concept, which has transformed the conventional SDLC model's concept of user–developer interaction into a three-dimensional model that includes developers, users and owners. Bhuvaneswari and Prabaharan (2013) discussed various SDLC models and gave suggestions, in particular situations, about what SDLC is best used in the developing project. They discussed the advantages and disadvantages of various models, such as the waterfall model, prototyping model, agile model, spiral model, iterative model, V model, rapid application development model and Big Bang model.

Despa et al. (2014) discussed various software development characteristics and gave the advantages and disadvantages of the various software development models. According to the authors, in any software development method, a proper development phase is the main aspect of the success of the software. It provides a formal software development methodology that helps in the innovation of the software industry. This paper shows the comparative study of different development methodologies and highlights their main characteristics. Dora and Dubey (2013) and Barjtya et al. (2017) discussed various software development life-cycle models in detail, such as the waterfall model, spiral model, agile model and V model. In these papers, the authors discussed some advantages and disadvantages of the above models. They also provided a comparative study between the agile model and other existing models. The authors said that the agile model helps to increase productivity and performance, and decrease time complexity and risk analysis. The authors also presented an overview of the agile model and discussed different agile development methods such as feature-driven development, extreme programming and crystal methods, etc.

The traditional model has a main focus on documentation and designing concepts of the software system. It follows the disciplines where the development of software is predictive and repeatable in nature. Hence, developers need more time and effort to develop the software and it is not able to solve the customer needs effectively. This is why the developer is attracted to another approach for constructing the software, and this advanced approach is based on the adapting nature. CBSE is an advanced approach where software is developed by selecting appropriate reusable components. The traditional approach does not focus on the reuse of software. The software is always built from scratch. Whereas, in CBSE, developers write code once and can reuse component code multiple times when needed. Therefore, the development cost and time for building large and complex software is minimized using this approach.

Chaudron et al. (2005) discussed the component-based development process and its life-cycle. According to the authors, the software development life-cycle model of components is different from the conventional life-cycle model. It contains two life-cycles that work simultaneously. They also discussed three other types of component-based development processes, such as product line development, architecture-driven component development and product line development. In this paper, the authors gave a comparative study between these three component-based development processes. With the help of a case study that is related to the software industry, it presents these three types of development processes, and uses different technologies and methods as needed. Capretz et al. (2004) discussed the life-cycle models based on component-based development and discussed various reusability issues that occur during any software product development. They discussed component-based process models in detail. This process model helps to increase reusability, evolution and productivity during the software development time. The authors also discussed some reusability techniques such as composition and inheritance that help to increase the software's productivity.

Fahmi and Choi (2008) discussed some life-cycle models based on component-based software development (CBSD), such as the Y model and V model. They also discussed some issues during the software development process, such as the CBSE life-cycle-related issue, the CBSE management issue, and trust and reliability on the component issue. The authors gave valuable suggestions to resolve the above issue effectively. Negi et al. (2015) and Gulia (2017) discussed various component-based software engineering models. They also compared all component models according to various parameters, such as domain analysis, component selection technique, risk analysis and component evolution for developing any software. According to the authors, in SDLC, a systematic arrangement of phases helps deliver high-quality software in good time. The authors also discussed the advantages and disadvantages of these different process models. Talukder and Rahman (2015) presented a comparative study between the different CBSD life-cycle models. They proposed a new life-cycle model called CROM (customer requirement-oriented CBSE life-cycle model). The proposed model handles the issue related to customers. It helps identify actual customer problems in developing software systems and maintain all customer demands through feedback analysis. This model increases the understanding between the customer and vendor for developing any software.

Khan et al. (2012) presented various characteristics of CBSD life-cycle models and proposed a new model called an improved model for reuse. This new model encompasses both component-based and software development processes. In this paper, the authors provided a comparative analysis between existing models with their proposed model and discussed their pros and cons. Garg and Jha (2019) compared various component-based life-cycle models and discussed a new proposed model that makes the component selection procedure easier. This proposed model provides the best-fit mechanism for the selection of any existing components. It contains three types of repositories, namely a black repository, white repository and gray repository. To construct any software, a developer can go to each repository in parallel and select appropriate components. Kaushik and Dulawat (2012) and Kumar and Bhatia (2014) discussed comparative analysis between the traditional life-cycle model and CBSD life-cycle models and described their strengths and weaknesses. According to the authors, the traditional approach only has limited requirements with limited features, but the component-based approach requirement changes frequently and supports design flexibility and reusability. According to the authors, component reusability is an emerging topic of the software engineering community. Reusability saves time and effort and reduces the development time and cost of software.

CBSE proposes an attractive approach that can be used to build any software application. This approach supports flexibility of design, changes requirements rapidly, improves quality and performance, and easily detects a fault in implementation (Nautiyal et al. 2012). Hence, due to these features, people get a better-quality product within time and budget. Due to the above facility, many IT industries are adopting this technology to develop healthcare software. In many healthcare applications, component-based approach is treated as a service-oriented approach that handles the complex environment software and gives a better analysis of the patient record (Chu 2005). Healthcare applications always insist on adopting best practices and software development, a process model that helps to improve the quality of care and fast recovery rate from the disease. Healthcare IT solutions help to improve interoperability between the doctor and patient, reduce the overall costs of healthcare delivery and increase the accessibility of patient records according to their requirement.

McMurtrey et al. (2013) discussed the impact of the component-based software development life-cycle model in the healthcare application. The authors also discussed various factors such as requirement analysis, design, risk analysis and select components for developing the healthcare application. In this paper, using an effective SDLC model, the authors designed and implemented a home health component with the help of pedagogical tools and this component can be used everywhere. According to the authors this home health software package provides the facility of regional hospital services.

The users' expectations are growing day by day, and the cost of a complex system is continuously rising due to this expectation. Hence, the developer feels pressure to provide more effective healthcare applications at a lower cost, with better quality, and safe and secure health services for the patient record. This is the reason the developer is shifting to develop healthcare software applications with specific advanced technology such as Blockchain that solves the problem related to healthcare applications. Healthcare software delivers secure data and enhances trust for both the doctor and the patient. Carroll et al. (2018) discussed the various challenges of the software engineering that is used in the healthcare industries, such as designing, dynamic processing, testing and deployment. According to the authors, software engineering plays an important role in many sectors, and healthcare application is one of them. In this paper, a new theory of software engineering related to healthcare software is introduced by the authors. They pointed out that better planning and balancing efforts deliver a safe and quality healthcare application. Lalband et al. (2019) discussed various modern software life-cycle models and represented how to implement smart healthcare applications using this model. According to the authors, systematic SDLC phases help to provide a high-quality healthcare application. Hence, healthcare always needs the best method and software development model. They also discussed the research challenges of software engineering for constructing a smart healthcare application.

Angraal et al. (2017), Bell et al. (2018), Katuwal et al. (2018), Ben Fekih et al. (2020) and De Aguiar et al. (2020) presented a survey of healthcare applications based on Blockchain. They discussed many applications in detail, such as electronic media records, pharmaceutical supply chain management, remote patient monitoring, health insurance claims, billing management, etc. They also discussed the limitation of healthcare applications based on Blockchain. They also pointed out some techniques that enhance the automation of medical services. According to the authors, Blockchain technology in healthcare applications can solve scalability, security and privacy issues. Blockchain technology removes the dependency of several mediators, decreases cost, and maintains trust and transparency. Siyal et al. (2019), Hasselgren et al. (2020) and Zhang and Boulos (2020) discussed the development of different healthcare applications using Blockchain technology. They pointed out some key elements such as interoperability, immutability transparency and decentralization of the Blockchain. They also discussed some use cases of

Blockchain that the various companies use. According to the authors, Blockchain provides safe and secure healthcare data management and increases reliability. Alla et al. (2018) discussed various features of the electronic healthcare system by using Blockchain technology. They represented a systematic review of healthcare software using Blockchain and found out the research gaps in the health sector. In this paper, the authors also discussed some advantages and disadvantages of adopting Blockchain technology in the healthcare sector.

9.3. Software development models

A software development process generally requires a framework that is used to analyze, plan, control and manage the process of software development. This framework is known as a software development life-cycle model (SDLC). An SDLC model is a systematic process for developing and designing a project from the beginning stage to completion (McMurtrey et al. 2013; Kneuper et al. 2017). A good software developer always chooses the best SDLC model based on the project context and user requirements for developing software. It provides a sequence of activities that helps to process, develop and maintain software products with improved quality and reliability. Different software life-cycle models may suit a project based on the user's requirement, cost, development time and project risks. In this chapter, we have discussed a comparative study of traditional software development life-cycle models, as well as modern software development life-cycle models based on component-based development. Traditional models do not support rapid changes in the requirements. They only focus on documentation rather than reliability or trust. In comparison, modern models handle these unwanted changes in the requirements successfully. They produce high-quality software in less time and maintain reliability and trust.

The basic software development model contains five states: requirement analysis, design, implementation, testing and deployment, as shown in Figure 9.3.

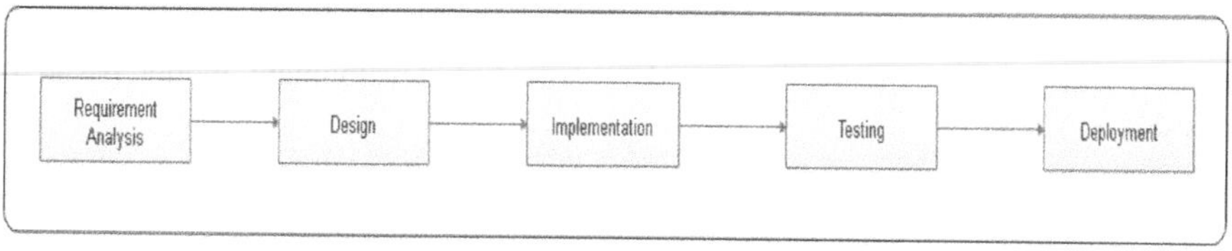

Figure 9.3. *Basic model for software development*

1) Requirement analysis: the first phase of developing software is the requirement analysis phase, in which developers analyze the need for software products according to the client. This phase collects detailed information about the desired product from the client and analyzes its functionality, development cost, technical issues, etc. After analyzing the desired product requirements, the developer prepares a document for the software product, which is called a software requirements specification (SRS).

2) Design: in this phase, the developer designs the basic structural framework of the software system. Developers decide what architecture and programming language are best for product development, which technology should be used, the constraints of the project, and how much time and budget should be used for developing software. This phase also decides how different modules of architecture communicate among them.

3) Implementation: in the implementation phase, developers actually start the development process according to SRS. This phase is also known as the building phase. In this phase, the developer follows all the standard guidelines of coding.

4) Testing: this phase is the last phase of SDLC before delivering the final software product to the customer. In this phase, the developer tests the final product, tracks where the bug is present in the implementation code and reports it. The testing phase confirms whether the final product meets the customer's requirement.

5) Deployment: once the software system is ready, the developer deploys this product for the user. In this phase, the developer releases the tested software products in the appropriate market. The developer releases their software products in a limited segment and analyzes their acceptance rate. After analyzing the acceptance rate, the product is released in a particular market based on the product's response.

In this chapter, we have given a brief comparative study of various software development life-cycle models and divided the software development life-cycle model into two categories. The first one is a traditional software development model, and the second one is a modern software development model based on CBSE.

9.3.1. *Traditional software development methodologies*

In this section, we have tried to illustrate some traditional software development models (Kaushik et al. 2012).

9.3.1.1. *Waterfall model*

The waterfall model is the first model, introduced by Royce in 1970 (Despa 2014). Another name for this model is a linear sequence life model, as all of the phases are executed one by one, as shown in Figure 9.4. Hence, the next phase starts only when the previous phase is fully executed. It does not allow us to go back to the previous step. It contains various phases, such as requirement analysis, system design, implementation, testing, deployment and maintenance (Kumar et al. 2014). The first phase in this model is the analysis of the requirements of the project. After analyzing, the next phase is the designing phase, in which the developer designs the framework of system according to the requirements and specifies the overall system architecture. After design, the next phase is the implementation phase, in which the design structure is translated into a programming language. After the development of the final product, the developers apply testing mechanisms, verify whether the product meets all of the user requirements or not, and detect faults and failures. The next step is the deployment phase, in which the product is deployed into the market for client use. The last phase is the maintenance phase. In this phase, the developer checks some issues after deploying the product in the client environment. If a problem occurs, they resolve that problem, increase productivity and release it. This model is used only for small projects and serves as a baseline for other models.

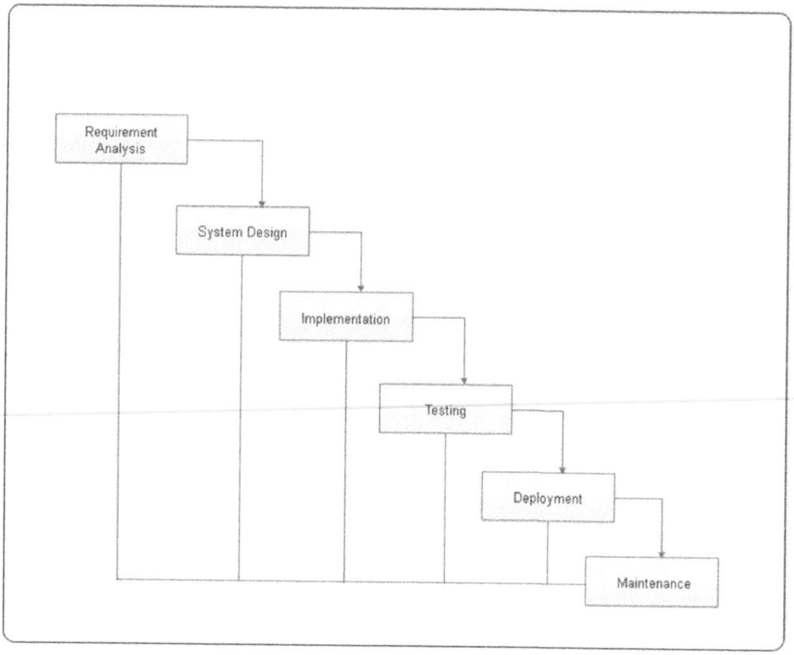

Figure 9.4. *Waterfall model for software development*

9.3.1.2. *Iterative model*

The iterative model is approximately similar to the traditional waterfall model, as shown in Figure 9.5. The traditional model follows the step-by-step process for developing a project, but the iterative model follows the cyclic process. The iterative model provides a feedback path in the preceding phase. After completing the project, developers can easily go back to the particular phase where an error has occurred. The feedback paths allow the reworking of the phase where the error was detected. This model contains various phases, such as requirement analysis, system design, implementation, testing, deployment and maintenance (Despa et al. 2014). The process of developing a project starts from a requirement phase. After collecting the product requirements from the client, the developer starts to design the project and finally implements the software product code on the basis of collecting requirements. After completing the coding, the developer applies some test methods to find an error. Once an error is detected, the developer goes back to that particular phase where the error occurred and corrects that error. At the end, it deploys the product in the client working environment. After deploying the product, if any bugs or errors are presented in the software, the developer updates the product with the help of a debugging process. This model is useful for small software applications.

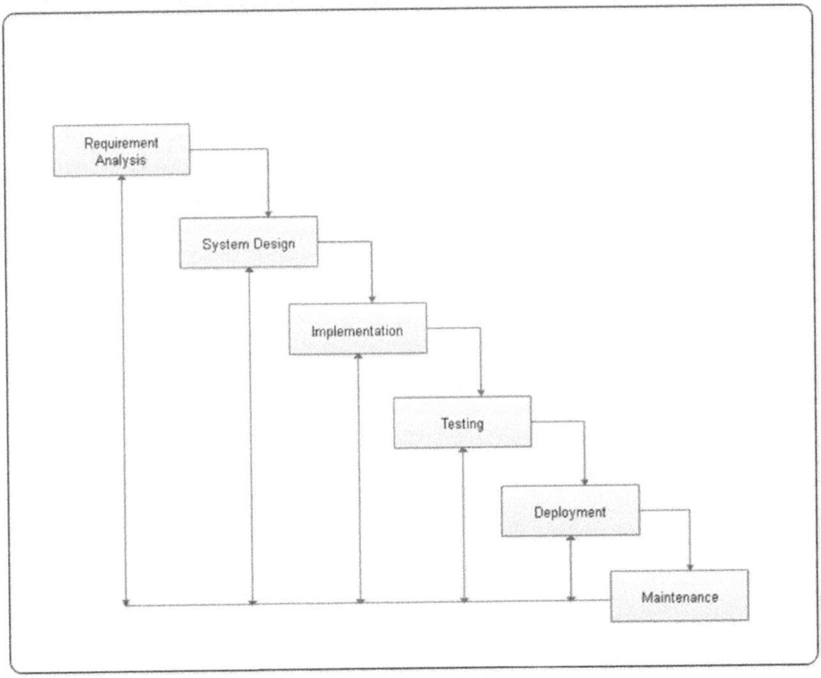

Figure 9.5. *Iterative model for software development*

9.3.1.3. *Prototyping model*

The prototyping model suggests that before developing the actual product, developers propose a working prototype of the software system (Despa et al. 2014). This model is used when the client does not know the exact requirement of the product and technical solutions are unclear to the developer. In this model, developers firstly develop a prototype of the product, then test and refine it on the basis of customer feedback. They repeat this process until the final acceptable prototype is achieved. After accepting the prototype, the developer designs, implements and tests the final product. This model contains various phases, as shown in Figure 9.6, such as requirement gathering, quick decision, build prototype, customer evaluation of prototype, refine requirements based on customer suggestions, design, implementation, test and maintenance. This model is useful in the absence of detailed information about the final product.

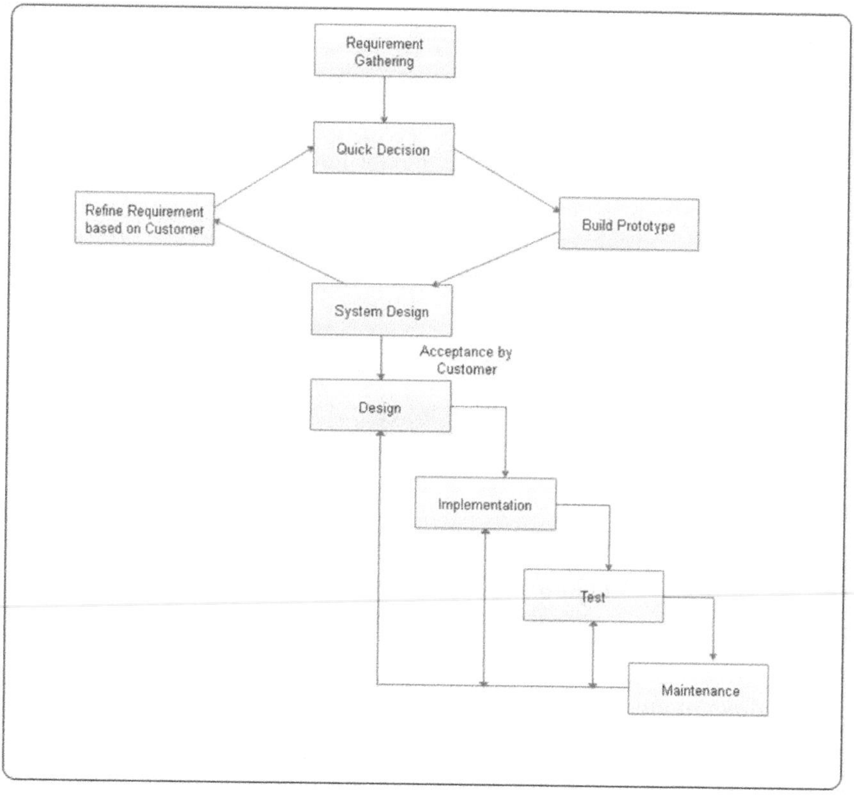

Figure 9.6. *Prototyping model for software development*

9.3.1.4. *Spiral model*

The spiral model is one of the most famous models of SDLC, as shown in Figure 9.7. The spiral model looks like a spiral with many loops. Each loop presents as a phase of a software process, such as determining objectives, identifying and resolving risks, development and testing, and planning the next iteration (Kumar et al. 2014). To develop the large and complex software, the spiral model is used in a real-time application. This model is helpful for reducing the risk factor of the project because it applies a risk reduction mechanism for analyzing risk at any stage. That is why it is known as a risk-driven process model. This model is used to build a high-quality product.

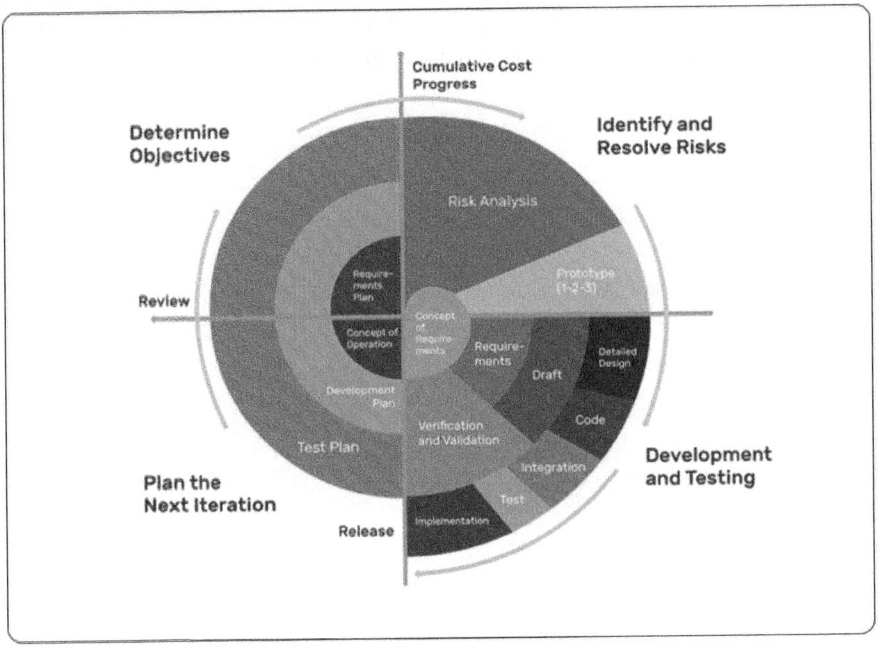

Figure 9.7. *Spiral model for software development (Kumar et al. 2014)*

9.3.1.5. *Agile model*

The agile model is based on the iterative development approach (Barjtya et al. 2017). In the agile model, the whole software project is divided into smaller iterations and each iteration is considered as a frame, as shown in Figure 9.8. This division helps us to minimize the risk factor of the project and reduces time and cost.

Each iteration goes through phases of the agile model, such as analyze, plan, design, develop, deploy and maintenance. This type of model is used when the customer needs more functional requirements with less time and effort. Hence, it gives more accurate, high-quality, flexible and reliable software products.

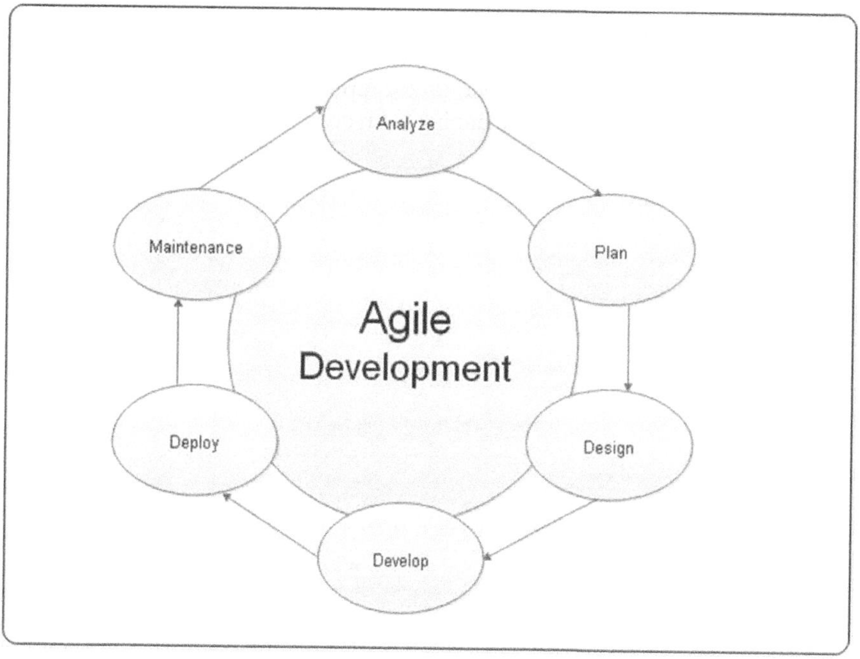

Figure 9.8. *Agile model for software development*

9.3.2. *Modern software development methodologies*

Some of the traditional models are based on a predictive approach, but the user needs to use the software life-cycle based on an adaptive approach. It must be flexible to accommodate the changing demands of the customer. Therefore, the developer moves to choose another modern software model that supports adaptive approach. In this section, we have discussed various component-based software development life-cycle models (Kaushik et al. 2012; Kumar et al. 2014).

9.3.2.1. *V model*

The V model is an improved model of the waterfall model, which is also called the verification and validation model (Chaudron et al. 2005). The verification phase exists on one side, and the validation phase exits on the other side, as shown in Figure 9.9. The verification stage locates model design with the help of requirement analysis. On the other hand, the validation phase checks the functionality and bugs with the help of testing. This type of model is suitable when the testing and deployment phases are run in parallel. This model is very useful, but it faces the difficulty that the developer never returns once the task is finished. Before developing the software, it is necessary to create a system test plan. This test plan is based on the functional requirement of the project. This model is suitable for large-scale projects where a lot of planning is involved.

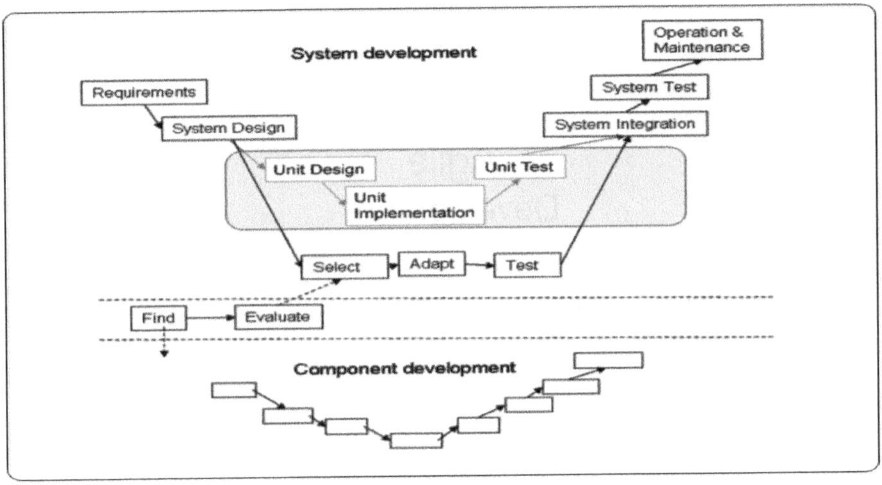

Figure 9.9. *V model for software development (Chaudron et al. 2005)*

9.3.2.2. *Y model*

Capretz et al. (2005) proposed the Y model. This model is based on a component-based development approach, as shown in Figure 9.10. The model's Y form makes it easier to iterate and overlap in appropriate places. Domain engineering, frame working, assembly, archiving, system analysis, design, implementation, testing, deployment and maintenance are some of the anticipated phases. This model supports change instability and the reusability concept for developing any software product. This model mainly focuses on software reusability during component-based development and emphasizes reusability when software is developed, evolves and desired reusable components are built on the assumption.

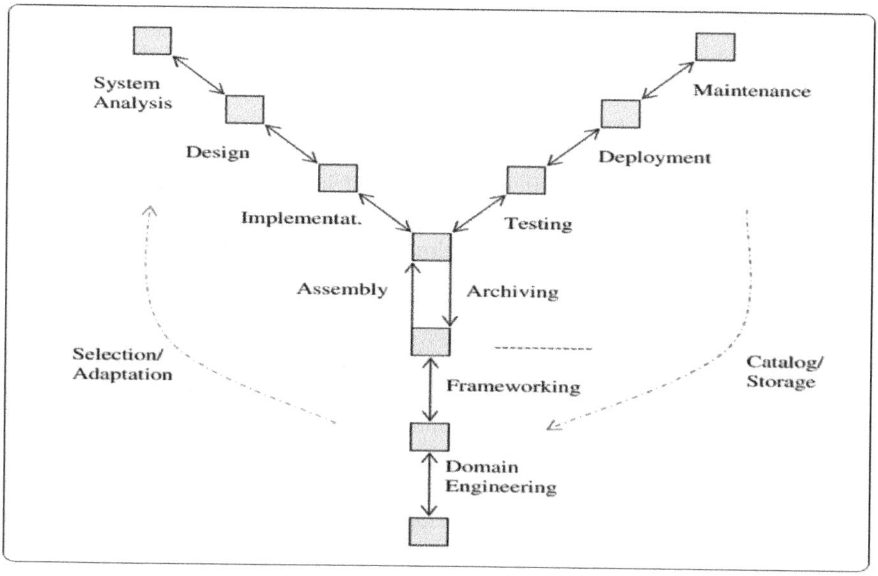

Figure 9.10. *Y model for software development (Capretz et al. 2005)*

9.3.2.3. *W model*

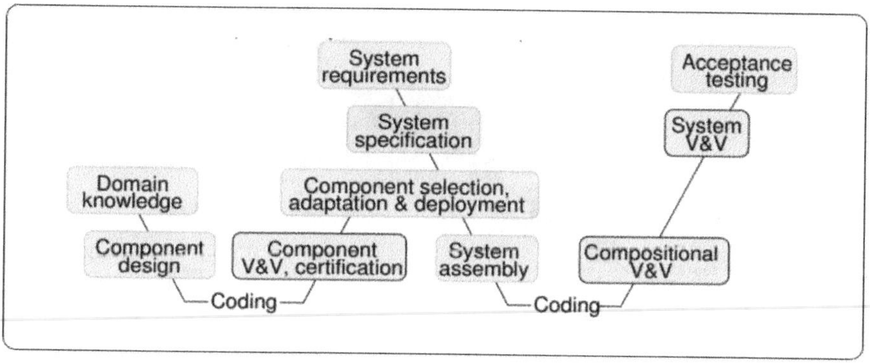

Figure 9.11. *W model for software development (Lau et al. 2011)*

This model is based on the V model, in which two V models are joined and work together, as shown in Figure 9.11. The first V model depicts the component life-cycle, while the second depicts the system life-cycle (Lau et al. 2011). The model is divided into two phases, one for component design and the other for component deployment. In the design phase, according to the domain engineering, software components are identified, designed and implemented. After building the component, it is stored in a repository, whereas in the deployment phase, the product is constructed and deployed using these already developed components.

9.3.2.4. *X model*

Tomar and Gill (2010) proposed the X model, which depicts how reusable components are used in complex and large-scale software projects. This model mainly focuses on reusability for developing software through the use of reusable components. As illustrated in Figure 9.12, the X model's life-cycle is divided into four sub-cycles: component-based software developer, development for reuse, development after modification and development without modification. This model supports the overlapping of different phases and increased complexity for developing any software.

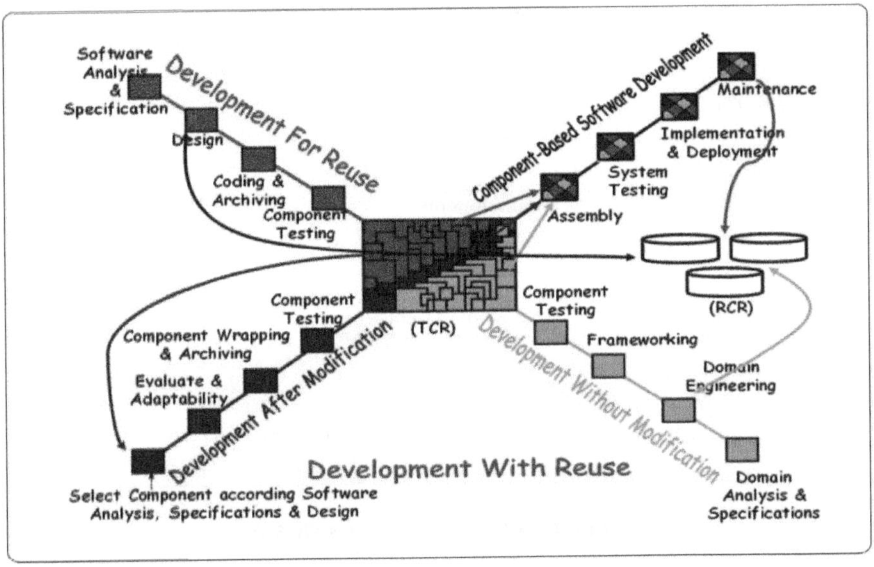

Figure 9.12. *X model for software development (Tomar et al. 2010)*

9.3.2.5. *An improved model*

Irshad and Noor proposed this model in 2012 (Khan and Khan 2012). In this model, the component development life-cycle and component-based system development life-cycle work in parallel, as shown in Figure 9.13. In this model, the authors discussed some issues related to component-based development and tried to reduce this issue by merging the traditional software development life-cycle model and component-based software development life-cycle model. This model helps us to resolve the problem related to unsatisfied requirements, repository management and the component's version handling.

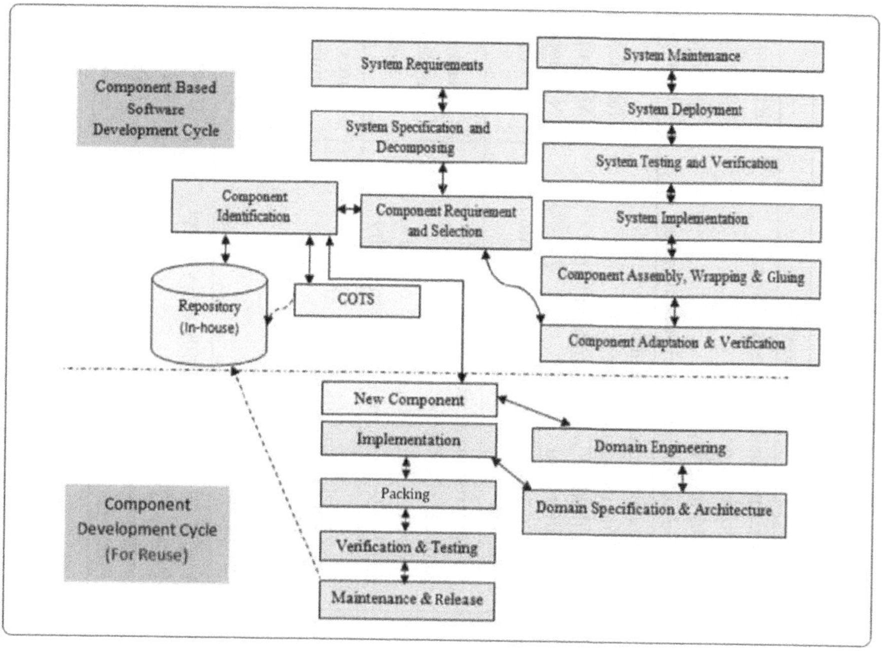

Figure 9.13. *An improved model for software development (Khan et al. 2012)*

Table 9.1 represents the comparison between different software development life-cycle models with their advantages and disadvantages.

Categories	Models	Advantages	Disadvantages
Traditional software development models	**Waterfall model**	– Simple and easily understandable – Easy to manage – Logical ordering – Simple planning and well-documented	– Risk involvement is high – Cannot go back to any stage after finishing – No accepted flexibility to change – No support for long-term project
	Iterative model	– Allows user to give feedback when the requirements are not clear – More flexible when compared to the Waterfall model – Emphasizes design over documentation of the project	– Iteration can be costly – More management is required – No support for long-term projects – Lack of proper documentation
	Prototyping model	– Accepts requirement changes rapidly – Reduces risk factor – Able to build a demo version of software – Easily identifies missing functionality	– Developer effort increases – Complexity of project increases – Implementation of prototypes is costly
	Spiral model	– Easy to plan and good negotiation – Supports risk management – Supports long-term project – Strong documentation	– More complicated compared to others – Requires high skill developers for analysis and planning – Can be a costly model – No support for small projects
	Agile model	– Understandable requirement document – Reduces this factor – Supports small project – Promotes maintainability	– Costly model – End requirement of project is not clear – Highly experienced people needed – Lack of proper documentation

Modern software development models	**V model**	– Supports component searching and retrieving method – Supports reusability of the component – Very simple and easy to understand – Risk involvement is low	– Project requirements unclear and ambiguous – Testing phase is not clear due to unclear requirements – It is a costly model – Very rigid and less flexible
	Y model	– Supports reusability – Supports both top down and bottom up approach – Supports component adaptation	– Overlapping and iteration occur during the process – Much effort is required to select the component – Component evolution is not possible
	W model	– Reusability is a key factor – Easily build a long-term project – Projects are more feasible	– Component evolution is not possible – Maintenance cost is high – Searching for a component technique is not effective
	X model	– Supports reusability – Provides clear requirements for the large project – Reduces cost and effort – Reduces risk factor	– Complexity increases for developing process – Development time and cost increases – Component evolution is not possible – Lack of proper risk analysis
	An improved model	– Supports reusability – Component evolution is possible – Easily possible component adaptation and selection	– No support for the certification process – No support for the trustworthiness property – Lack of scalability

Table 9.1. *Advantages and disadvantages of various SDLC models*

9.4. Proposed model

The healthcare industry has grown over the past few years, and software technology plays an important role in the evolution of the healthcare sector. Healthcare is one of the most rapidly growing industries that connects many fields directly, physically, emotionally, mentally and financially. The technology related to healthcare faces many challenges: it needs advanced medical devices; it has not used a proper methodology for developing the software system; it requires clinics; rising medical care costs, etc. All of these challenges affect the quality of medical care. So, it requires an advanced business model for healthcare technology that maintains a proper standard for developing any software in which people may trust support. Many healthcare policies help the best software practices and design principles to secure it (Lalband et al. 2019). In developing any healthcare software system, cost, time, effort, trust and security are the main factors that affect the development process. An effective SDLC helps to reduce these kinds of difficulties. SDLC is defined as a framework based on the project context and is helpful for producing high-quality software. Better life-cycle model-based software improves the quality of care of the patient record. Hence, for better-quality healthcare software used for tracking and processing patient information effectively. It reduces manpower requirement and treatment costs, and easily accesses patient information on time (Katuwal et al. 2018; De Aguiar et al. 2020).

Traditional models do not have better support to develop large and complex software, and hence, fail to provide better quality and accuracy. Therefore, the developer chooses another advanced SDLC model technique that solves the above issues. This advanced SDLC model technique is based on CBSE, in which software systems are developed by selecting reliable and reusable components, and assembling them together with the suitable software architecture. This new approach is different from the conventional approach, where software is not developed from scratch. It consists of two life-cycles that work in parallel, one is a component-based development life-cycle and another one is a system development life-cycle through components (Kaushik et al. 2012; Kumar et al. 2014). This approach increases the software's productivity and performance, but does not increase its reliability and trust due to the selection of software components, which are not always trustworthy and reliable. Hence, the developer needs to better software development life-cycle with advanced technologies such as Blockchain, cloud computing, AI and IoT that increase the reliability and trust in them (Angraal et al. 2017; Bell et al. 2018).

In the proposed method, we have looked at the impact of the healthcare sector using a new technology called Blockchain. Blockchain is one of the technologies that can be used to secure our data and increase our trust in any application. This technology is becoming popular because of its features such as security, decentralization, immutability and transparency. In this chapter, we have developed a component-based life-cycle model using Blockchain technology and created a Blockchain-based repository that stores software components in the form of blocks. Using Blockchain-based software, we try to keep a patient record in the form of a block, which can be made available securely, and only to authorized users. The doctors may easily access and store the medical history of the patients anytime and anywhere. Hence, this type of software product increases the patient's trust, and this data cannot be misused by unauthorized persons. Figure 9.14 represents a detailed overview of our proposed life-cycle model. The detailed description of the proposed model based on component-based software engineering via Blockchain technology is given below.

The life-cycle of CBSE is different from the traditional way of developing software. It works simultaneously through two development life-cycles, namely a component development life-cycle and a component-based software development life-cycle.

9.4.1. *Component-based software development life-cycle*

The software development life-cycle with components includes all the activities of the software system's production. In this cycle, the software system is built by using pre-existing components that are stored in a repository. Software developers reuse these components according to the requirement of their applications. It contains the following phases: requirement, system specification, component search and selection, component identification, component adaptation, system implementation by assembling the component, system testing and verification and system deployment, as shown in Figure 9.14. The first phase is the requirement phase, in which all the initial requirements of the users are identified. The developer understands and identifies these requirements for a particular application. After collecting the requirements, the developer analyzes the feasibility of the component on the basis of the requirements. In this phase, the developer also studies the software application's constraints, functional and non-functional requirements, and prepares a document for the requirement specifications of the system.

In the next step, developers search and select the desired components in an internal reusable repository using various searching techniques (such as keyword-based, faceted, enumerated, attribute value, signature-based techniques, etc.). If the required components are not available in the repository, then the developer needs to implement components via Blockchain technology. Using the component development life-cycle, the developer creates a component in the form of a block, stores it in a Blockchain-based component repository and provides proper indexing. In this phase, the developer decides which component should be reused and should be built from scratch using the system requirements for building the software system. The next phase is the component identification phase, in which the developer identifies the target component and selects the component that satisfies the needs of the software system being developed. Domain engineering (product line engineering) is helpful in this phase. The next phase is the component adaptation phase. After selecting the candidate component, some of the selected components may not fit as per the specifications required by the software. There may be a gap between the component features and features required from the component by the system architect. The component adaptation techniques (such as component wrapping, coordinate, adaptation pattern) help to minimize these mismatches between the component required and component available. In the next phase, if the verified component fits their specific system requirement, then the developer composes the software through these verified components. After constructing the system through the composition of the component, the next phase is system testing and verification. In this phase, the system requirements should be matched with the final implemented system. In this step, the developer follows some standard testing and verification techniques. The developer also checks undesirable effects and errors in the software application. In the last phase, the final software product is delivered to the customer for its use. Before reaching the customer, this product is well examined and corrected for faults, and the adaptation of the system in a changing environment is confirmed.

9.4.2. *Component development life-cycle*

When a component is not found in the repository, the developer creates a new component from scratch, as shown in Figure 9.14. The life-cycle of component development contains the following phases: domain specification of the component, implementation of the component as a block, testing and verification through the consensus algorithm, deployment of the component, component code storage and indexation. The first phase is the domain specification of the component. It provides the information from the domain knowledge of the new component to build a software system. This phase helps the developer to understand the domain knowledge of application and systematic component reuse. After understanding the domain specification of the component, the developer develops a component according to system requirements. This phase aims to develop a component in the form of a block via Blockchain technology. The developer considers every component as a block in Blockchain, and the block is linked by a cryptographic hash. To create a component, the developer firstly initializes the genesis block. It is the first block in the Blockchain to which the other blocks are connected. Then, it creates a new block that stays connected to the genesis block. This new block divides into two parts. The first part is the header that stores the index of the block, timestamp and proof of work. The second part stores the component's data. Here, the data is stored in JSON format. The data part contains various attributes, such as language, processor, operating system, functionality, version, domain and hash code file of the component. These attributes help in the selection and storing of components from the Blockchain repository. The hash code of the file, in which the component developer writes the component's code, is generated using the Interplanetary File System (IPFS).

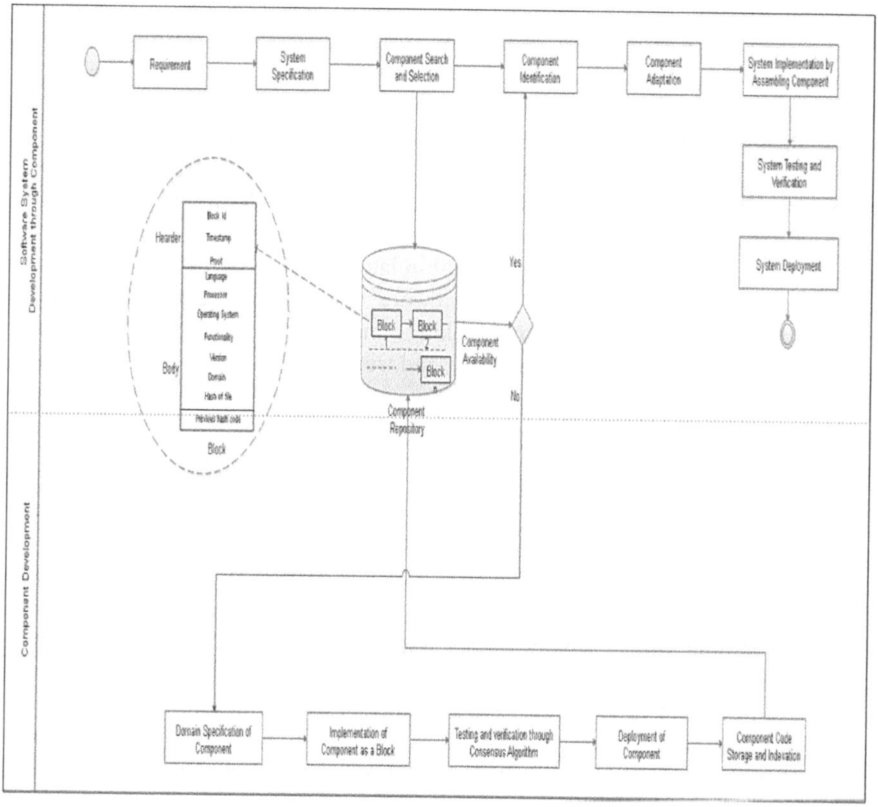

Figure 9.14. *Proposed method*

After implementing the component as a block, the next phase is the verification and testing phase. In this phase, the developer mines the newly created block by using a consensus algorithm. Mining of a block is a process to verify a new block (component). The developer uses a consensus algorithm called the proof of work that is maintained by all participants for the verification and validation of blocks. A consensus algorithm is used to select a leader (miner), who will decide the content of the next block. After verification, the new block is added to the Blockchain. The next step is the deployment of the component. In this phase, new components are assembled into a package that is capable of distribution and installation. These components are tested and are also ready to be deployed in any environment. In the final phase, the new components are stored in a repository to build the software through component composition in the future. The developer assigns some indexes to the components for easy retrieval from the repository.

9.5. Comparison among different software development life-cycle models

In this section, we have presented a comparison among different life-cycle models for software development. Table 9.2 lists the comparative analysis of various software models with our proposed model. It clearly shows that by using the software development life-cycle model we have proposed for developing healthcare software, the developer ensures that health-related data are secure, increases trust in data and improves the quality of healthcare applications. Hence, better-quality healthcare software is used for tracking and processing patient information effectively. It decreases manpower hours and treatment costs, and can access patient information easily and on time.

9.6. Conclusion and future works

In this chapter, we have discussed how software systems affect healthcare applications. The healthcare software has changed the human lifestyle and plays an essential role in human life and behaviors. It provides many facilities, such as effective learning, utility, saving money, increasing productivity and controlling it. Systematic software development has been used to improve patient care and secure health record effectively. It provides a common understanding for processing the software building. Hence, healthcare applications need to adopt advanced technology with an effective life-cycle model based on Blockchain. It improves the quality of care, reduces processing costs and most importantly, enhances care efficiency, an increased trust in data. It also effectively maintains and updates medical records. The primary objective of this chapter is to provide a systematic component-based life-cycle model with advanced technology such as Blockchain. It provides a perfect development process and understanding, which affects the quality of the healthcare service. Component-based healthcare software is able to eliminate all kinds of healthcare inefficiencies and problems. In future work, we will work on a formal aspect of the proposed model.

Characteristics	Waterfall model	Iterative model	Prototyping model	Spiral model	Agile model	V model	Y model	W model	X model	An improved model	Proposed model
Requirement analysis and specification	In the beginning	In the beginning	In the beginning	In the beginning	Frequently changed	Frequently changed	Frequently changed	Frequently changed	Frequently changed	Frequently changed	Frequently changed
Project cost	High	High	High	High	High	Low	Low	Low	Low	Very low	Very low
Project development	Long	Long	Long	Long	Long	Short	Short	Short	Short	Very short	Very short
System verification and validation	At the end	At the end	At the end	In some stage	In some stage	In some stage	In every stage	In every stage	In every stage	In every stage	In every stage
Documentation	Very simple	Very simple	Very simple	Simple	Understood	Understood	Well understood	Well understood	Well understood	Well understood	Well understood
Long-term management project	No	No	Partially supported	Partially supported	Yes	Partially supported	Yes	Yes	Yes	Yes	Yes

Scalability support	No	No	No	No	Partially supported	Yes	Yes	Yes	Yes	Yes	Yes
Overlapping phases	No	No	Yes	No	No	Yes	Yes	Yes	No	No	No
Maintenance	Less	Less	Less	Less	Considerable	Less	Considerable	Considerable	Considerable	Support maintainability	Support maintainability
Risk analysis	No	Limited	Limited	Yes	Yes	Limited	Yes	Yes	Yes	Yes	Yes
Reliability	No	No	No	Limited	Yes	Yes	Yes	Yes	Yes	Yes	Yes
Reusability	No	No	No	No	No	Limited	Yes	Yes	Yes	Easy to achieve	Easy to achieve
Evolution support	No	No	No	No	No	No	No	No	No	Partial	Yes
Certification support	No	No	No	No	No	No	No	No	No	Partial	Yes
Trustworthiness support	No	No	No	No	No	No	No	No	No	Partial	Yes

Table 9.2. *Comparative analysis of various software models with our proposed model*

9.7. References

Alla, S., Soltanisehat, L., Tatar, U., Keskin, O. (2018). Blockchain technology in electronic healthcare systems. *IIE Annual Conference. Proceedings*, 901–906. Institute of Industrial and Systems Engineers (IISE).

Angraal, S., Krumholz, H.M., Schulz, W.L. (2017). Blockchain technology: Applications in health care. *Circulation: Cardiovascular Quality and Outcomes*, 10(9), e003800.

Aoyama, M. (1998). New age of software development: How component-based software engineering changes the way of software development. *1998 International Workshop on CBSE*, 1–5.

Barjtya, S., Sharma, A., Rani, U. (2017). A detailed study of software development life cycle (SDLC) models. *International Journal of Engineering and Computer Science*, 6(7), 22097–22100.

Bell, L., Buchanan, W.J., Cameron, J., Lo, O. (2018). Applications of Blockchain within healthcare. *Blockchain in Healthcare Today*, 1. DOI: 10.30953/bhty.v1.8.

Ben Fekih, R. and Lahami, M. (2020). Application of Blockchain technology in healthcare: A comprehensive study. *International Conference on Smart Homes and Health Telematics*, 268–276. Springer, Cham.

Bhuvaneswari, T. and Prabaharan, S. (2013). A survey on software development life cycle models. *International Journal of Computer Science and Mobile Computing*, 2(5), 262–267.

Cai, X., Lyu, M.R., Wong, K.F., Ko, R. (2000). Component-based software engineering: Technologies, development frameworks, and quality assurance schemes. *Proceedings Seventh Asia-Pacific Software Engeering Conference, APSEC 2000*, 372–379, IEEE.

Capretz, L.F. (2004). Software process model for component-based development. *Information Technology Journal*, 3(2), 176.

Capretz, L.F. (2005). Y: New component-based software life cycle model. *Journal of Computer Science*, 1(1), 76.

Carroll, N., Kuziemsky, C., Richardson, I. (2018). Special issue on software engineering for connected health: Challenges and research roadmap. *Journal of Software: Evolution and Process*, 30(7), e1941.

Chaudron, M., Larsson, S., Crnkovic, I. (2005). Component-based development process and component lifecycle. *Journal of Computing and Information Technology*, 13(4), 321–327.

Chu, S.C. (2005). From component-based to service oriented software architecture for healthcare. *Proceedings of 7th International Workshop on Enterprise Networking and Computing in Healthcare Industry, HEALTHCOM 2005*, 96–100, IEEE.

De Aguiar, E.J., Faiçal, B.S., Krishnamachari, B., Ueyama, J. (2020). A survey of Blockchain-based strategies for healthcare. *ACM Computing Surveys (CSUR)*, 53(2), 1–27.

Despa, M.L. (2014). Comparative study on software development methodologies. *Database Systems Journal*, 5(3), 37–56.

Dora, S.K. and Dubey, P. (2013). Software development life cycle (SDLC) analytical comparison and survey on traditional and agile methodology. *National Monthly Refereed Journal of Research in Science & Technology*, 2(8), 22–30.

Fahmi, S.A. and Choi, H.J. (2008). Life cycles for component-based software development. *2008 IEEE 8th International Conference on Computer and Information Technology Workshops*, 637–642.

Gajalakshmi, P. (2016). Software development lifecycle model (SDLC) incorporated with release management. *International Research Journal of Engineering and Technology*, 3(4), 1536–1543.

Garg, K. and Jha, S.K. (2019). Component based life cycle models comparative survey. *2019 2nd International Conference on Power Energy, Environment and Intelligent Control (PEEIC)*, 23–26, IEEE.

Gulia, P. (2017). Component based software development life cycle models: A comparative review. *Oriental Journal of Computer Science and Technology*, 10(2), 467–473.

Hasselgren, A., Kralevska, K., Gligoroski, D., Pedersen, S.A., Faxvaag, A. (2020). Blockchain in healthcare and health sciences – A scoping review. *International Journal of Medical Informatics*, 134, 104040.

Katuwal, G.J., Pandey, S., Hennessey, M., Lamichhane, B. (2018). Applications of Blockchain in healthcare: Current landscape & challenges. arXiv preprint arXiv:1812.02776.

Kaushik, M. and Dulawat, M.S. (2012). A comparision between traditional and component based software development process models. *Journal of Computer and Mathematical Sciences*, 3(3), 248–421.

Khan, A.I. and Khan, U.A. (2012). An improved model for component based software development. *Software Engineering*, 2(4), 138–146.

Kneuper, R. (2017). Sixty years of software development life cycle models. *IEEE Annals of the History of Computing*, 39(3), 41–54.

Kumar, G. and Bhatia, P.K. (2014). Comparative analysis of software engineering models from traditional to modern methodologies. *2014 Fourth International Conference on Advanced Computing & Communication Technologies*, 189–196, IEEE.

Lalband, N. and Kavitha, D. (2019). Software engineering for smart healthcare applications. *International Journal of Innovative Technology and Exploring Engineering*, 8(6S4), 325–331.

Lau, K.K., Taweel, F.M., Tran, C.M. (2011). The W model for component-based software development. *2011 37th EUROMICRO Conference on Software Engineering and Advanced Applications*, 47–50, IEEE.

Mahmood, S., Lai, R., Kim, Y.S. (2007). Survey of component-based software development. *IET Software*, 1(2), 57–66.

McMurtrey, M. (2013). A case study of the application of the systems development life cycle (SDLC) in 21st century health care: Something old, something new? *Journal of the Southern Association for Information Systems*, 1(1).

Nakamoto, S. (2009). Bitcoin: A peer-to-peer electronic cash system [Online]. Available at: https://bitcoin.org/en/bitcoin-paper.

Nautiyal, L., Tiwari, U.K., Dimri, S.C., Koolagudi, S.G. (2012). Component based software development – New era with new innovation in software development. *International Journal of Computer Applications*, 51(19), 5–9.

Negi, D., Chauhan, Y.S., Dimri, P., Harbola, A. (2015). An analytical study of component-based life cycle models: A survey. *2015 International Conference on Computational Intelligence and Communication Networks (CICN)*, 746–750, IEEE.

Ragunath, P.K., Velmourougan, S., Davachelvan, P., Kayalvizhi, S., Ravimohan, R. (2010). Evolving a new model (SDLC Model-2010) for software development life cycle (SDLC). *International Journal of Computer Science and Network Security*, 10(1), 112–119.

Rastogi, V. (2015). Software development life cycle models-comparison, consequences. *International Journal of Computer Science and Information Technologies*, 6(1), 168–172.

Siyal, A.A., Junejo, A.Z., Zawish, M., Ahmed, K., Khalil, A., Soursou, G. (2019). Applications of Blockchain technology in medicine and healthcare: Challenges and future perspectives. *Cryptography*, 3(1), 3.

Talukder, S.C. and Rahman, M.M. (2015). Customer requirements oriented component based software development life cycle model. *2015 International Conference on Computers, Communications, and Systems (ICCCS)*, 61–68, IEEE.

Tomar, P. and Gill, N.S. (2010). Verification & validation of components with new x component-based model. *2010 2nd International Conference on Software Technology and Engineering*, 2, V2–365, IEEE.

Ullah, H.S., Aslam, S., Arjomand, N. (2020). Blockchain in healthcare and medicine: A contemporary research of applications, challenges, and future perspectives. arXiv preprint arXiv:2004.06795.

Vale, T., Crnkovic, I., De Almeida, E.S., Neto, P.A.D.M.S., Cavalcanti, Y.C., de Lemos Meira, S.R. (2016). Twenty-eight years of component-based software engineering. *Journal of Systems and Software*, 111, 128–148.

Zhang, P. and Boulos, M.N.K. (2020). Blockchain solutions for healthcare. *Precision Medicine for Investigators, Practitioners and Providers*, 519–524. Academic Press.

10

The Role of Smart Contracts and Blockchain Technology in Healthcare and Other Use Cases

Newly emerging technologies have encouraged every sector to adopt these technologies to increase their productivity. The traditional techniques have been replaced by digital techniques to overcome the limitations faced by the people. One of the emerging technologies is Blockchain technology, which offers multiple benefits to business enterprises. The smart contract is a Blockchain-based technology that overcomes the limitation experienced in traditional contracts. This chapter explains the concept of a smart contract and its role in different sectors in detail. The research begins with the introduction of smart contracts, moving forward to its challenges, the real-time companies using smart contracts, with some past historic attacks. Overall, this chapter's research consists of deeper knowledge about smart contracts, their platform and real-time applications.

10.1. Introduction

The evolution of technologies has unboxed tremendously easier and simpler applications. These applications have turned the traditional approaches into smarter ones. A similar example is a Blockchain-based technology known as "smart contracts" (Rouhani and Deters 2018). Emerging technologies have reduced the effort needed and saved a lot of time. The term smart contract came into existence to overcome the limitations faced in traditional contracts. A traditional contract is defined as a bunch of agreed-upon terms between two parties that are validated and signed by the two parties. Smart contracts replace the issues that occurred in traditional contracts. There are a few similarities as well as dissimilarities between smart contracts and traditional contracts (Toshev & Boteva 2020). The traditional

Chapter written by Abhishek BHATTACHARYA, Tanupriya CHOUDHURY and Roohi SILLE.

contract systems are enforced by the law and agreed upon thoroughly by both parties. But the major difference is that traditional contract is based on natural human language, whereas smart contracts are based on digitally signed laws (IBM n.d.; Infosys n.d.; Investopedia 2022). There are multiple differentiating factors. These differences are as follows.

10.1.1. *Comparison between traditional contracts and smart contracts*

10.1.1.1. *Automated contract*

It takes more time to prepare, draft and formulate a traditional contract. Usually, it takes around one to three days to prepare the contract. Smart contracts need more time to code the contract. Smart contracts are time-consuming to develop but once deployed the contracts are automated. There are ready-made platforms present like Ethereum, Hyperledger Fabric, etc., that automate contracts.

10.1.1.2. *Contract remittance and execution*

In traditional contracts, some obligations are applied to the parties to pay the overdue within the allocated time as an organizational effort. Whereas in smart contracts, the remittance of the contract is executed automatically once the contract is fulfilled. These values and statements are recorded in the form of code (Toshev & Boteva 2020).

10.1.1.3. *Low cost*

In traditional contracts, the procedure fee is slightly higher as lawyers, contract makers and other third parties are involved. Smart contracts preferably require less cost.

10.1.1.4. *Data security and confidentiality*

Traditional methods may not maintain the security and confidentiality of the data. Traditional contracts require paperwork that opens the door for entering threats. However, smart contracts enable a strict path for data security and confidentiality. They use Blockchain-based cryptographic protection to maintain the confidentiality and integrity of data.

10.1.1.5. *Physical presence*

In traditional contracts, the two parties must be present physically; without their presence, the contract cannot be signed and it is impossible to proceed. In this ever-changing world, smart contracts are signed digitally anywhere and the contracts can be accessed anytime.

10.1.1.6. *Archiving*

Traditional contracts require more space, time, administration and supervision, which results in a lengthy procedure. Smart contracts follow a secure and automated procedure that avoids time consumption and the usage of natural resources (Toshev & Boteva 2021).

The above-mentioned points differentiate traditional contracts and smart contracts with definite parameters. In the next section, we provide detailed information about Generation Two of Blockchain – Ethereum.

10.2. Ethereum: Generation Two of Blockchain technology

Blockchain (Khanna et al. 2021; Sah et al. 2021) developers have thought of creating a simpler interface for smart contracts compared to existing ones. The newly emerged second generation of Blockchain (Khanna et al. 2020a, 2020b), known as Ethereum, was evolved to ideate assets that would add more benefits to Blockchain technology. Initially, to define Ethereum, it is a decentralized open-source platform that enables smart contract functionality. After Bitcoin, the second-largest evolution of cryptocurrencies in the market is Ethereum. Its evolution took place in 2013 by the programmer Vitalik Buterin. This Blockchain technology had a boost in 2014, with a supply of 72 million coins in the beginning. This platform permits the developers to build and operate tasks that users rely on for interaction (Corporate Finance Institute n.d.; NTU 2020).

Ethereum is defined as the public open-source Blockchain platform that enables the functionality of smart contracts and is another leading platform in the cryptocurrency market with a secured environment (Corporate Finance Institute n.d.; NTU 2020). Ethereum holds specifically two accounts, one is an externally owned account and the other is a contract account. The externally owned account can be controlled with the help of a private key.

10.2.1. *History of Ethereum*

The founder of Ethereum, Vitalik Buterin, was first a Bitcoin programmer in 2011; he initially worked for Bitcoin Magazine. Later, he realized some other platforms that can bring a distinct view towards Blockchain technologies. In 2013, Ethereum was established as a general scripting language (NTU 2020; Corporate Finance Institute n.d.). In 2014, the team at Ethereum launched a campaign where they sold Ethers to check how it affects the world. At the same time, they raised 80 million dollars (Corporate Finance Institute n.d.; NTU 2020).

10.3. Smart contracts

In 1996, a smart contract was defined as a digital contract structured in the form of lines of code and executed in the same way. It is a set of protocols formed between parties to fulfill the desired promises. The smart contract executes the contract, ensuring no malicious contents as well as unpredictable circumstances. It reduces the usage of third parties, which results in low transactional cost, and lowers potential collusions and countered risk. Smart contracts came into existence due to Blockchain technologies (Wang et al. 2019). They are in the form of general-purpose programming. These lines of code and the agreements are stored over distributed and decentralized technology termed as Blockchain.

The specialty of smart contracts is that they are reliable and trustworthy, and permit a faster flow of procedure without any involvement or interference from third parties, or the legal systems. Smart contracts are stored over Blockchain technology that runs on preferred conditions (Wang et al. 2019). Smart contracts are solely focused on automating the execution of the agreement without any loss of time or certain involvement. Users develop their code and form a Turing complete program on the Blockchain network.

Smart contracts are developed on the Ethereum platform. The execution of text on Ethereum consists of the heap, stack and a determined memory over the chain. Once the development of the contract is accomplished, the next step is to deploy the contract. After the deployment of the contract, the contents of the contract cannot be changed or altered, even by the contract creator. The execution of a contract requires a set of operations and specified functions to be carried out. Once the set of functions is carried out, then the program can be finished by the gas depletion. In the next section, we explain the term gas in detail.

10.3.1. *How smart contracts work*

Smart contracts follow a stipulated model and are entirely executed on the Blockchain. A contract is transformed into lines of code that are then executed under certain conditions. A wide range of networks execute the actions over the set of protocols that are verified and validated. The actions related to smart contracts are conducted and executed. These actions involve vehicle registration, notifying the users, raising a ticket and transferring funds to relevant parties. These chunks of actions, once executed, are updated on Blockchain, and mark the transaction as completed. To dive deeper, a smart contract is more than a general script or piece of code that is stored on a decentralized Blockchain network. It maintains transparency between the two parties. Importantly, smart contracts contain terms and conditions in the form of code that helps participants to clearly understand the contract signing digitally, without any enforcement of laws or any legal mechanism (Kemmoe et al. 2016).

Smart contracts are surrounded by a cryptographic protection. The presence of cryptographic protection confirms that the contents of contracts cannot be altered at any cost. It follows a strict security path ensuring the backup of contracts. Smart contracts have multiple benefits, which are as follows.

10.3.2. *Benefits of smart contracts*

1) Speed: smart contracts are a digital contract which means that the tasks are automated once the action is executed. It speeds up the procedure because it reduces paperwork (IBM n.d.; Infosys n.d.; Investopedia 2022).

2) Efficiency: smart contracts are effective as well as efficient. This is because they are packaged in a secure environment and do not involve hectic legal procedures. The best part is that there is no need for physical presence at the time of signing the agreement (IBM n.d.; Infosys n.d.; Investopedia 2022).

3) Accuracy: smart contracts maintain the accuracy of the contents, ensuring that the same task is performed without any misconception or errors, whatever the action (IBM n.d.; Infosys n.d.; Investopedia 2022).

4) Trusted and transparent: people usually avoid digital techniques because of insecurity and lack of trust. But this is not the case with smart contracts. The strict cryptographic protection locked the contract into a safe network where there is no possibility of threat or alteration. The contracts are visible and accessible to parties connected with the network (IBM n.d.; Infosys n.d.; Investopedia 2022).

5) Security: security is the strength of a smart contract based on Blockchain technology. Firstly, any contracts contents stored over Blockchain networks are encrypted. The hacker cannot attack the network. If the hacker attacks the network, it will have to change the entire chain of records as the contents are stored over the distributed ledger (Investopedia 2022).

6) Cost-effective: smart contracts are an automated procedure that executes actions without the usage of paper. This reduced the cost spent on paperwork as well as its fees for overall procedures (IBM n.d.; Infosys n.d.; Investopedia 2022).

10.3.3. *Roles of smart contracts*

Smart contracts may change to deal with various activities like transactions or any other legal work. For enterprises, organizations and institutions, it may be difficult to deal with so many contracts, store them in files and then act accordingly. Smart contracts play a vital role in various sectors, providing them with the flexibility to independently handle contracts without any burden of storage, or spending time as well as money on paperwork (Salmerón-Manzano and Manzano-Agugliaro 2019).

Smart contracts have made it feasible for businesses and trade to anonymously identify the parties without any intervention of a middleman. Smart contracts have reduced the cost usually required for traditional contracts without affecting authenticity and integrity (Salmerón-Manzano and Manzano-Agugliaro 2019). Therefore, smart contracts are useful in various sectors, such as travel companies, supply chain deals, logistics deals and many others. Smart contracts enable features that help both parties to easily carry out their work in an isolated secured environment.

10.4. Use of smart contracts in healthcare, patient monitoring, and other use cases

By now, we are well aware of how critical smart contracts can come to be when certain functionalities are concerned – and many of these completely deal with decentralization as the core concept (or for the matter of absence of centralization) for certain processes, procedures and use cases. The concept of smart contracts, though first introduced by Ethereum, which also marked the onset of Blockchain technology's second generation, actually helped shape the development of similar technologies across other platforms and products. Currently, there are many public as well as consortium Blockchain implementations that provide support for writing and deploying smart contracts, and many times it is in a different language than what Ethereum supports. This has given rise to many developers being able to write smart contracts in languages that they knew before they started in the domain of Blockchain technology – such as Java, JavaScript, Rust, etc.

As more and more engineers become equipped to write smart contracts, the total number of use cases that can see the usage of smart contracts is increasingly growing. When such a turnout happens before and during an ongoing pandemic, it brings out several use cases that are concerned with the domain of healthcare. This can specifically encompass patient monitoring, vaccination drives, vial information, supply chain management of medical equipment, vaccines, medicines and electronic health records (EHRs), further securing protected health data/information (PHI) and regulated access to patient information, as well as ailment data. As healthcare is a massive industry in itself, the use cases that it encompasses usually see a lot of complexity. The same can be said about the deployments trailed on the back of smart contract technology.

However complicated it may sound to build new applications, platforms and functionalities on the new-age technology called Blockchain using concepts further next-gen such as smart contracts, it is indeed quite straightforward to implement certain use cases, at least in the shape of a PoC (proof-of-concept). Below are some of the implementations and deployments being carried out by multiple organizations across the globe, either as PoCs, SaaS (software-as-a-service)-based offerings or fully-fledged deployments connected to legacy systems.

10.4.1. *Transparency in supply chain*

A significant challenge in the healthcare sector is to confirm the authenticity of medical devices. Blockchain becomes the centerpiece while companies try to streamline their supply chains to allow themselves, as well as customers, to track items throughout the chain. This results in complete transparency across the value chain.

This has been a big reason to worry about the fact that counterfeit drugs cause tens of thousands of serious ailments and even deaths every year.

Main benefits of Blockchain in such use cases:

– Compliance: it is imperative to be able to record and report elements in a supply chain. Combining supply chain data in a single system helps optimize compliance.

– Customer trust: it is important for medical device and drug manufacturers to be able to build trust with their customers. Doing so is increasingly possible by tracking the products using a Blockchain, which includes third-party integrations with manufacturers, distributors, etc.

10.4.2. *Electronic health records on the Blockchain*

Health systems across the globe face the issue of information being restricted to data silos, thus leaving patients, as well as hospitals, with an incomplete picture of health records forming their medical history.

A valid solution would be to put these EHRs (Electronic Health Records) on a Blockchain-based system, which will eventually give a complete picture regarding a patient – depending on the kind of access privileges. Such access, as well as data additions, can be managed using hashes inserted into the Blockchain, and the patient can provide approval for sharing such data typically by signing these transactions on the Blockchain network.

In such a case, every change to the records and instance of patients' approval to share their medical record is committed as a transaction on the Blockchain.

Blockchain-enabled EHRs have many benefits. Health insurers can receive validated confirmation of health services directly and instantly from the patient without the expense of an intermediary. As an example, Medicalchain is developing a platform on which other digital health solutions can be built, which include virtual counselling services and medical data exchange, enabling patients to sell their anonymized medical records and data in exchange for MED tokens to help them develop digital health applications.

10.4.3. *Use of smart contracts for insurance and billing in supply chain management*

Many providers offer Blockchain-based systems that allow various healthcare players, such as pharmaceutical companies, wholesalers, insurers and healthcare providers, to verify their corporate identity, log contract data and track transactions of goods and services, and payment processing data for these goods and services. By sharing digital contracts between manufacturers, retailers and healthcare organizations, instead of each player having their own version of contracts, they can significantly reduce disputes over quality checks, chargebacks, claims and other issues.

10.4.4. *Verification of medical personnel's identity cards*

Verifying background information has been an important cause across domains. When it comes to healthcare, institutes need to be certain about the experience of a medical professional.

US-based company ProCredEx has developed such a system for verifying medical certificates using the R3 Corda Blockchain protocol.

The main advantages of the Blockchain system in such a use case are:

– faster approval from health institutes and hospitals during the recruitment process;

– transparency and security for partners and vendors, for example, organizations outsourcing representatives, or in new virtual care models to inform patients about the experiences of medical staff.

10.4.5. *IoT security for remote patient monitoring*

What we can also see all around us these days is the use of smart devices to monitor our health – fitness bands, weight trackers or even a ring that can monitor your health, sleep and activity patterns, such as the Oura ring. Talking about the medical devices at large, hospitals and institutes have started employing multiple IoT-based devices to track the health of a patient constantly. This may include the elderly who need constant supervision, even while discharged from hospitals.

In such scenarios, the security protocols followed by these devices become a high priority, and the use of Blockchain to successfully trace any intrusions is a good starting point. Additionally, permissioned Blockchains would ensure that only approved nodes (devices) can interact with the system.

10.5. Building smart contracts on the Ethereum Blockchain

Ethereum Blockchain is the second-largest cryptocurrency available on the market, after Bitcoin. The evolution of Ethereum had brought significantly great success since its establishment in 2015. The invention of a Russian Programmer conveniently lead to new decentralized applications to be developed. For the development of decentralized applications, Ethereum is the best Blockchain platform recommended. To create your contracts, you can reliably use the Ethereum Blockchain platform. Ethereum is a distributed infrastructure that potentially assists in accomplishing projects. Smart contracts can be created, developed and deployed using Ethereum Blockchain (NTU 2020). You can create smart contracts on the Ethereum platform, so let us understand the execution procedure involved in execution in detail.

10.5.1. *Ethereum virtual machine (EVM)*

EVM is a virtual machine acting as a runtime environment for building smart contracts on the Ethereum platform. EVM is sandboxed from the host operating system. Each EVM runs when any single contract is executed. Smart contracts prefer the Ethereum platform for deployment because of its higher abstraction layer. It is the global supercomputer that gears up the execution of every action. EVM does not make any delayed Internet calls or pass on any random number as it is solely a virtual machine. EVM prefers programming language coding compared to assembly language (NTU 2020; SitePen 2020). Some components take part while implementing the smart contracts on the platform. Each component is explained below in detail.

Before that, we have mentioned a summary of the working of smart contracts on Ethereum. Smart contracts that need to be developed on Ethereum prefer to use code in the solidity programming language. Once the program is written, it is compiled into bytecode because EVM understands bytecode easily. Then, this bytecode is deployed in the Ethereum network transaction. Ethereum depicts the value of a token called Ether (Yuan et al. 2018). Ethereum supplies operations including computation and data transfer with a fixed price. Also, only the desired amount of gas is consumed that is needed for the execution of the operation. The transaction contains a term named gas limit that means to define maximum gas consumption. After the contract calls the function, it requires the lower limit of gas to be specified. There are some conditions applicable during execution (Yuan et al. 2018). If the function executes normally, then it uses the corresponding gas and returns the leftover gas (Yuan et al. 2018). This is the standard procedure while deploying the smart contract on Ethereum.

10.5.2. *Gas*

Gas is a measuring unit present inside EVM to allocate particular fees for each transaction within smart contracts. Every action of computation needs a certain amount of gas. The more the computation is, the more gas is used. Now, to program on Ethereum, a specific programming language called Solidity is needed.

10.5.3. *Solidity*

Solidity is the programming language defined for smart contracts developed on Ethereum. On the top layer of Ethereum, smart contracts are developed using Solidity, which is a simple object-oriented programming that uses class or language. Solidity does not have a difficult syntax that is tough to understand (SitePen 2020). This programming language is influenced via popular languages that developers prefer. These are C++, Python, JavaScript. It can perform several arbitrary computation activities like raising tickets, sending and gaining tokens, and core operations.

To build smart contracts on Ethereum, the initial prerequisites are mentioned. For instance, let us create a cell phone contract (SitePen 2020). This contract solely lies between the company and the subscriber. The steps follow the procedure to create a cell phone contract (SitePen 2020):

1) create a theory-based cell contract using Solidity;

2) use a function to define the structure of the contract;

3) add the company functions as well as the subscriber functions within the code;

4) compile and run the code;

5) finally, test the code to check whether the contract is working fine.

10.6. Real-time use cases of smart contracts

Smart contracts have multiple use cases in various industries, but the ultimate use cases where the role of a smart contract is reflected are mentioned below.

10.6.1. *Smart contracts and insurance*

For insurance companies, it is difficult to manage several contracts conducted between the customers and the company. These contracts contain terms and conditions that need to be signed by both parties. The core requirements focus on the insurance claim, reimbursement of expenses and renewal of insurance. These industries are looking for an automation solution that reduces paperwork, invites events and activates the agreement. Smart contracts in insurance industries handle the entire procedure of insurance, beginning from the claim of policy or executing automated actions as per the agreement. Smart contracts settle the payout efficiently. These insurance contracts are hard-coded ones that cannot be altered later due to strict security (Grasso 2019; IONIXX 2018).

10.6.2. *Smart contracts in an electric vehicle*

Sooner or later, smart contracts will be used in the transport or automotive sectors. Due to high rates of fuel, electric vehicles will be preferred most. These electric vehicles are associated with IoT sensors, and smart contracts so that the recharge of electric vehicles becomes faster. Smart contracts provide flexibility to business processes so that the users can securely make the payments to recharge their electric vehicles (Grasso 2019).

10.6.3. *Smart contracts in the energy sector*

The flow of energy depends on the act's decentralization, decarbonization and digitalization. The energy consumers, as well as the energy producers need turning energies that can upgrade more resources. Therefore, energy sectors are even looking for advancement to secure their resources and make them faster. Smart contracts play a vital role in defining the distributed energies as per the agreed terms. Smart contracts even facilitate easy integrations with IoT devices (Grasso 2019).

10.6.4. *Intellectual property rights*

Smart contracts play a vital role in several sectors. One of these sectors is intellectual property rights. Using smart contracts, artists, music directors and television shows can easily protect their content and apply copyrights over them. For instance, a music director deals with a party that needs to reform their song. In that case, the music director can create certain protocols, paying high royalties, and protecting information about the project. These clauses can be set together using smart contracts. Thus, smart contracts protect intellectual property rights (Grasso 2019; IONIXX 2018).

10.6.5. *Stock trading*

The market fluctuates every moment; hence, the traders are looking for some autonomous transactions that cost less and are less time-consuming. Smart contracts contribute in every sector just to automate the task. Similarly, smart contracts even help to record every movement of the stock or follow it once it is transferred to its owner. The traders can buy or sell their stocks quickly because the smart contracts update the transactions. Before updating the transactions, it records and validates the transactions automatically (IONIXX 2018).

Several companies are present that prefer to use smart contracts to track the records and source positive outcomes for their business. Below, we have mentioned in detail some specific companies that are using smart contracts on a real-time basis.

10.7. Six companies using smart contracts in real-world applications

10.7.1. *Slock.It*

Slock.It has changed the look of the sharing economy and how it works. This is possible only because of smart contracts. It automates the procedure of payments or sharing documents and rentals. Recently, the company Slock.It worked with Share & Change, acting as a helping hand to provide a sharing rental payment service. Therefore, the company Share & Change uses smart contracts to pay rent to use electric vehicles. Depending upon the requirements, Slock.It has made universal network sharing, which is an open-source network that deploys Blockchain modules. Once done with the deployment, the third-party companies can add their services or products to this network (PolySwarm 2018).

10.7.2. *Fizzy AXA*

The French Airline AXA built flight insurance over the Blockchain platform. AXA ideated a simple way that benefits a wide range of travel insurers. It is difficult to work with airline companies that are crediting compensations for late flights. Whether it is flight travel insurance or the reason for the delay of a flight, it is the biggest challenge to get compensation without any delay. Fizzy AXA was initiated to resolve this problem. It outsources specific conditions that can be applied for compensations. Fizzy says that if a flight is delayed for more than two hours, this information is loaded onto the app, then the desired compensation is credited directly to the bank account. This contemporary feature is possible only because of smart contracts. Here, the use of smart contracts is made by setting some parametric insurance, where users are not allowed to take compensation for the total loss, rather than compensating the traditional loss. This flight insurance is based on a triggering action, which is the flight being delayed for two hours. This condition is only available for flights between the U.S and Paris, even with an extended plan till 2018. To avail these products, it is mandatory to pay a subscription fee (PolySwarm 2018).

10.7.3. *Etherparty*

Etherparty is one of the leading startups. They are referred to as "The Smart Makers". This tech startup permits users to build their smart contracts on the platform. Etherparty contains the wizard of contracts and holds around 500 pre-registered users who can access uncountable templates of contracts. It has designed the templates elegantly, so that users do not need prior knowledge about smart programming to create a contract. The users have the flexibility to create several kinds of contracts, such as peer-to-peer escrow contracts, tokens, real estate agreements, Supply Chain contractor's agreements and additionally, any other contract based on any domain. Etherparty assures the company about the quality of the product. It ensures that the company adopts the technologies easily, escalating processes and mitigating risk (PolySwarm 2018).

10.7.4. *Propy*

Smart contracts play a crucial role in the real estate sector, where several properties are discussed between the buyers and sellers. One of the companies took the initiative to bridge the gap between the buyers and sellers by introducing smart contracts. Propy is one of the premium leading companies that started using smart contract techniques in the real estate sector. It initiated the first transaction in

September 2017 that ranged around $60,000 in Ukraine. This big marketplace provides flexibility to the buyers and sellers, as well as brokers for listing out properties across the borders. Once finalized with the property, the buyers and sellers actively participate in smart contracts ensuring fair and legal norms. For instance, the buyer selects a property and is willing to purchase it. Thus, the buyer decided to reserve the property, paying an initial token of a certain amount. But then if the seller denies selling the property, then due to smart contracts, the token amount is credited back to the buyer's account. The smart contract facilitates the entire paperwork procedure, and signatures can be provided remotely via an app (PolySwarm 2018).

10.7.5. *Populous*

The business gets its amount from unpaid invoices in the form of invoice financing. The process involves beginning with the invoice buyers paying for the invoice of business and then giving back the original amount once the debitter repays it. Populous took the opportunity to replace this present scenario and instead use smart contracts. Populous made it feasible to purchase and sell the required outstanding invoices over the Blockchain platform using smart contracts. Smart contracts have benefited the business in various fields, resolving its limitations. It speeds up the process, but considers factors like mitigating risks, involvement of manual human error and replication of invoice financing. Populous overcomes the above factors, executing the tasks automatically. For instance, once the invoice is uploaded by the seller along with terms and conditions, the buyer has to select the finance amount option and the rest of the transactions will be done automatically. These amazing features encourage leading businesses and startups to approach smart contracts (PolySwarm 2018).

10.7.6. *PolySwarm*

Out of the several marketplaces, PolySwarm is one of the leading decentralized threat intelligence marketplaces. The involvement of smart contracts even facilitated the threat intelligence marketplace. Business organizations post their security issues that need to be resolved. They reward the person who resolves the security issues with accuracy. The role of smart contracts adds some automation. The security expert who resolves the threats with accuracy receives the reward automatically without any manual activities. Thus, smart contracts brought innovation in the cybersecurity domain, sourcing more effective solutions.

To sum up, the above list depicts the companies who worked with smart contracts in real life and even received positive outcomes. Smart contracts promise to automate all of the transactions without the involvement of manual work. Although smart contracts are time-consuming in the development phase, once they are deployed, the activities turn into faster automation (Medium 2021).

10.8. Challenges

Building smart contracts gives rise to multiple benefits, but simultaneously there are some challenges to be addressed while using smart contracts based on Blockchain technology:

– Confidentiality: although Ethereum promises to deliver transparency, enterprises still hesitate to store their contracts publicly because of competitive strategies. Ethereum does not support private smart contract Blockchain platforms that can harm confidentiality.

– Inception to human error: the smart contracts are formatted in lines of code, but there may be a possibility that the terms and conditions related to transactional data may be affected because of missed code. This can decrease accuracy and reliability.

– Threats through bugs or errors: in 2016, because of a vulnerability in the smart contracts of the DAO, 50 million ETH was siphoned off by hackers. This resulted in the fork of ETH into ETC (Ethereum Classic).

– Predictability: smart contracts automate depending on the event that is triggered. Depending on the parameters set, the smart contracts perform certain actions. For instance, let us consider, the stock price's multiplication factor fluctuates, which is not in the control of the smart contract; this may result in certainly unplanned contract code executions.

– Correctness: one of the major challenges faced while using smart contracts is that once the smart contract is developed and deployed, it cannot be altered. Any error can be exploited.

– Scams: as Blockchain is a newly emerging technology, it may be vulnerable to malicious attacks and threats. Therefore, these vulnerable attacks can be initiated through scams or honeypots.

10.9. Historical attacks and issues with smart contracts

Previously, smart contracts were prone to various security issues and attacks. The most discussed attacks are the DAO attack and the Parity Wallet hacks. These were the two historical attacks that took place, impacting smart contracts negatively. DAO is a smart contract that permits people to exchange their tokens and win rewards. In 2016, DAO gathered a fund of 150 million USD. Participants can buy tokens and vote over prepositions, receiving rewards. Later, it was affected by several threats that created loopholes and removed funds. The hacker attacked the smart contracts, which gave way for vulnerability to enter in the form of bugs or errors in the code (Sayeed et al. 2019).

Another historical popular attack took place at Parity Multisig Wallet. This was discovered when the hacker had an opportunity to make the wallet vulnerable with version 1.5+. This flaw allowed the hacker to remit more than 30 million USD, which is around 150 million Ether. Once the Parity Wallet initiated a smart contract, two hacks took place consecutively. The attacker executed a script that used bugs. Due to this, two hacks were initiated; in the first one, the attacker initiated a call to update the status of the wallet. This means the attacker can act as an owner and remove all of the funds from the wallet (Sayeed et al. 2019).

10.10. Conclusion

Smart contracts are hassle-free digital contracts that do not have any intervention from third-party lawyers or legal enforcement. This seamless technology can be built using the Ethereum Blockchain platform, which provides security through cryptographic and encryption algorithms. A cyber-attack cannot directly hit a single record, as Blockchain is a chain of records that is connected with a global supercomputer network. This chapter describes the use cases, benefits and challenges of smart contracts. Smart contracts even have multiple benefits that can minimize all the disadvantages faced while dealing with traditional contracts. But since the technology acts as a boom and even a curse, smart contracts are similarly leading to cyber threats and cyber-attacks, which can create loopholes and vulnerabilities that can cause harm. In this chapter, we have mentioned the six ultimate companies that had implemented smart contracts on a real-time basis. The results indicate that the companies experienced a positive impact using smart contracts. Smart contracts do not involve the intervention of a middleman or any legal person. Instead, smart contracts reduced the transactional cost and manual work. Implementing smart contracts takes time, but once the smart contracts are deployed, they automatically fulfill the set of promises mentioned in the smart contract. Apart from the numerous benefits and features of smart contracts, the developers may come across some other challenges. To sum up, smart contracts have several advantages, but simultaneously need to answer some challenging questions. Still, if businesses prefer smart contracts with strict security protocols, then it is one of the best-recommended Blockchain-based technologies.

10.11. References

Alharby, M. and van Moorsel, A. (2017). Blockchain-based smart contracts: A systematic mapping study. *AIS, CSIT, IPPR, IPDCA*, 125–140.

Agarwal, A. (2021). Smart contracts: Challenges advancements, platforms and applications [Online]. Available at: https://www.linkedin.com/pulse/smart-contracts-challenges-advancements-platforms-ankit-agarwal/ [Accessed 17 August 2021].

Arc Touch (2018). How to be smarter about developing smart contracts in solidity [Online]. Available at: https://arctouch.com/blog/how-to-develop-smart-contracts/ [Accessed 17 August 2021].

Choudhury, T., Khanna, A., Toe, T.T., Khurana, M., Nhu, N.G. (eds) (2021). *Blockchain Applications in IoT Ecosystem*. Springer International Publishing, Cham.

Clack, C.D., Bakshi, V.A., Brain, L. (2016). Smart contract templates: Foundations, design, landscape and research directions. arXiv:1608.00771v3.

Corporate Finance Institute (n.d.). What is a smart contract? [Online]. Available at: https://corporatefinanceinstitute.com/resources/knowledge/deals/smart-contract/ [Accessed 17 August 2021].

Grasso, A. (2019). Smart contracts: Real-life use cases [Online]. Available at: https://antgrasso.medium.com/smart-contracts-real-life-use-cases-f1dd03a76d5 [Accessed 17 August 2021].

Hu, Y., Liyanage, M., Manzoor, A., Thilakarathna, K., Jourjon, G. (2019). Blockchain-based smart contracts – Applications and challenges. arXiv:1810.04699v2.

IBM (n.d.). What are smart contracts on blockchain? [Online]. Available at: https://www.ibm.com/in-en/topics/smart-contracts [Accessed 17 August 2021]

Infosys (n.d.). Smart contracts: Introducing a transparent way to do business [Online]. Available at: https://www.infosys.com/insights/digital-future/smart-contracts.html [Accessed 17 August 2021].

Investopedia (2022). Smart contracts [Online]. Available at: https://www.investopedia.com/terms/s/smart-contracts.asp [Accessed 17 August 2021].

IONIXX (2018). Examples of smart contracts in the real world [Online]. Available at: https://blog.ionixxtech.com/4-examples-of-smart-contracts-in-the-real-world/ [Accessed 17 August 2021].

Kemmoe, V., Stone, W., Kim, J., Kim, D., Son, J. (2016). Recent advances in smart contracts: A technical overview and state of the art. *IEEE Access*.

Khanna, A., Sah, A., Choudhury, T. (2020a). Intelligent mobile edge computing: A deep learning based approach. *International Conference on Advances in Computing and Data Sciences*, April, 107–116. Springer, Singapore. DOI: 10.1007/978-981-15-6634-9_11.

Khanna, A., Sah, A., Choudhury, T., Maheshwari, P. (2020b). Blockchain technology for hospitality industry. *European, Mediterranean, and Middle Eastern Conference on Information Systems*, November, 99–112. Springer, Cham. DOI: 10.1007/978-3-030-63396-7_7.

Leeway Hertz (n.d.). Steps to create, test and deploy Ethereum smart contracts [Online]. Available at: https://www.leewayhertz.com/ethereum-smart-contract-tutorial/ [Accessed 17 August 2021].

NTU (2020). Writing smart contracts in Ethereum Blockchain [Online]. Available at: https://www3.ntu.edu.sg/home/ehchua/programming/blockchain/ethereum.html [Accessed 17 August 2021].

PolySwarm (2018). Companies already brilliantly using smart contracts [Online]. Available at: https://medium.com/polyswarm/5-companies-already-brilliantly-using-smart-contracts-ac49f3d5c431 [Accessed 17 August 2021].

Rouhani, S. and Deters, R. (2018). Security, performance, and applications of smart contracts: A systematic survey. *IEEE Access*.

Sah, A., Negi, D., Rawat, S., Choudhury, T., Khanna, A. (2021). Block chain platforms and smart contracts. *Blockchain Applications in IoT Ecosystem*, 65–76. Springer, Cham. DOI: 10.1007/978-3-030-65691-1_5.

Salmerón-Manzano, E. and Manzano-Agugliaro, F. (2019). The role of smart contracts in sustainability: Worldwide research trends. *MDPI*, 11(11), 3049.

Sayeed, S., Marco-Gisbert, H., Caira, T. (2019). Smart contract: Attacks and protections. *IEEE Access*.

SitePen (2020). Smart contracts: A tutorial [Online]. Available at: https://www.sitepen.com/blog/smart-contracts-a-tutorial [Accessed 17 August 2021].

Toshev & Boteva (2020). Main differences between traditional contracts and smart contracts [Online]. Available at: https://www.toshevboteva.com/publications/main-differences-between-traditional-contracts-and-smart-contracts [Accessed 17 August 2021].

Wang, S., Ouyang, L., Yuan, Y., Ni, X., Han, X., Wang, F.-Y. (2019). Blockchain-enabled smart contracts: Architecture, applications, and future trends. *IEEE Transactions on Systems, Man, and Cybernetics: Systems*, 49(11), 2266–2277.

Yuan, R., Chen, H.-B., Zang, B.-Y. (2018). ShadowEth: Private smart contract on public Blockchain. *Journal of Computer Science and Technology*, 33(3), 542–556. DOI 10.1007/s11390-018-1839-y.

11

Healthcare Research Using Blockchain Technology: A Future Perspective

Blockchain has expanded from the cryptocurrency world to the medical field. The significant issues associated with handling the volume of data present in the medical industry are also addressed by this technology, in addition to security. The processing of vast amounts of data and security are the industry's two biggest challenges. In terms of handling electronic health records, medical personnel credentialing, IoT-enabled healthcare monitoring, counterfeit pharmaceuticals, managing pharmaceutical supply chains, etc., Blockchain has offered a fantastic solution. In each of these areas, Blockchain can be of great help to the medical sector. This study examines how Blockchain technology is being used in the aforementioned categories of the healthcare industry and the difficulties encountered.

11.1. Introduction

The enormous economic sector that deals with data processing, analysis and other data-related activities is the healthcare sector. Because it can handle massive amounts of data and analyze it effectively, Blockchain technology has greatly improved the medical industry. The processing of vast amounts of data and patient data security are two issues that medical data must address. A group of computers that are not owned by a single company administer a time-stamped collection of permanent data records known as a Blockchain. This data is organized into blocks that are connected to one another and protected by cryptographic principles (e.g. chain). Blockchain technology has received a great deal of attention because it offers cryptographic security for data distribution, meaning that no one can decode the encrypted data after it has been disseminated throughout the network. Since the healthcare industry has to do a lot to maintain the confidentiality of data, merging

Chapter written by Bhumika SHARMA, Roohi SILLE and Tanupriya CHOUDHURY.

the healthcare industry with Blockchain can handle and transfer vast amounts of data. Blockchain can help medical professionals not only safeguard electronic health information, but also keep track of patient progress and monitor their health in real time. The combination of Blockchain and AI can quickly assist doctors and radiologists to fully analyze the patient's body and make health predictions for the patient.

The healthcare sector has benefited greatly from Blockchain in terms of the security of electronic medical records, the performance of maintaining data transparency, which is the most crucial factor when dealing with medical health records, and secure data transmission in the form of data clusters.

11.2. Benefits of using Blockchain in the healthcare industry

The healthcare industry may be significantly impacted by Blockchain. With regard to patient data transparency and future development execution, this technology could help medical specialists and other industry professionals (Dagher et al. 2018). A variety of Blockchain setups can also be specifically tailored to serve various use cases in the healthcare sector. Among other things, this list includes the secure administration of electronic health records (EHRs), drug traceability, patient consent management, data security in clinical preliminary studies (Benchoufi et al. 2017) and support via micropayments. The contact and costs of existing delegates can be reduced thanks to the healthcare prospects of Blockchain. To improve access to and segment the value of care, the environmental stakeholders have teamed up with innovation. Faster access to clinical records leads to longer-lasting improvements in health.

– The ability to fully secure each patient's EHR. The management of numerous records and reports that are categorized and subject to strict regulations is a common practice in the healthcare industry. One such statute is the 1996 Health Insurance Portability and Accountability Act (HIPAA). Most often, these entries are stored in a single database, which can cause interoperability and security problems (as was the case in the first section) (Cai and Zhu 2016; Kiyomoto et al. 2017).

– Ease to trace the patient's health by tracking their records. Here, we use smart contracts innovation to achieve constant, consistent traceability with pop-up messages to limit human mediation and subsequent undesired postponements.

– At the moment of transmission, maintain the security of medical data. The development of systems to ensure security and protection is necessary for Blockchain innovation, just like for other types of innovation that can hold data. Because Blockchain data is stored publicly and shared by all members, the majority of cryptographic operations anticipate keys to enable those cryptographic processes; this necessitates some level of encryption/access control.

11.3. Application of Blockchain in the healthcare industry

Let us talk about the various use cases of Blockchain in the healthcare industry. Starting with the pharmaceutical industry, security and stability are given the highest priority. Blockchain implementation can improvise supply chain management monitoring and recording by reducing the scope for human error and delays. By keeping track of the products to prevent the flow of falsified drugs in the market, which can lead up to $200 billion loss, the products can be verified. Many big companies have already taken advantage of this technology to have more effective solutions. Some of these companies are Blockpharma, Chronicles and Modum. The proposed solution is the creation of a sensor that keeps track of the physical conditions that the product goes through. These records are permanently stored on the Blockchain for future reference.

DNA data, also called genomic data, is an entirely new market that requires Blockchain security. The secure exchange of genomic data can be empowered with the assistance of a Blockchain organization. As this is a developing business sector, there are many use cases that can emerge from assortment, stockpiling and examination using Blockchain. This market alone could cost billions of dollars. What makes Blockchain a fitting choice here is its decentralization, permanence and transparency properties. Clinical records and data are significant and straightforward, and approved clients have continuous access to the latest treatment data (Mettler 2016). In addition, there are data avoidance methods that give protection, traceability and respectability to the common data. Furthermore, patients are generally mindful of who is accessing their data (Yue et al. 2016).

The healthcare and financial areas are in conflict over the installments to be made in the healthcare areas. The installments made for patients and their families for operations, trading of clinical gear and compensation installments are just a few of the instances of cost associated with healthcare. It is miserable to say that our health industry is experiencing an outdated healthcare installment process, in which thousands of dollars are squandered due to the failure of the installment framework. Blockchain has decentralization properties; it allows financial transactions and resource tracking to record every value. Blockchain with decentralized properties additionally guarantees the verification of other confidential data and records stored in blocks along the Blockchain (Sullivan and Burger 2017). The normal list allows individuals to progressively screen and break down the assets engaged from the beginning to the end (Pouraghily and Wolf 2019). The present critical problem area is the process that enables the security of the whole system, the pre-authorization process, which includes some insurance organizations that are expected to decide earlier whether to pay for explicit organizations. Concluding a certain financial amount is covered by a part's insurance contract that enters a languid cycle for certain reasons, for example, the commitment of different accomplices in the adjustment of the total covered. Considering the payer–provider relationship, the cycles are generally puzzling, incorporate a couple of manual advances and may be a direct result of sad correspondence and development. With Blockchain, a singular record split between the clinical consideration accomplices consists of the patient's honor and splendid arrangements used for the pre-authorization process. This motorizes data combination and trading, taking into account continuous confirmation of benefits. Some of the benefits of incorporating Blockchain integrate further, creating pay for faster trade settlement, helpful patient treatment, exact portions to the provider, lower administrative costs and twofold record-keeping. Given that the quantity of healthcare transactions is monstrous, a special advancement of the Blockchain is expected. The final test is a 51% assault. Although this is only a hypothetical gamble, an unmistakable arrangement should be proposed (Ahram et al. 2017).

Independent experts known as "smart contracts" are stored in a Blockchain technology and work to encrypt and transform transactions into contracts or authoritative documents in order to provide legitimate sorts of aid (Anjum et al. 2017). These smart contracts include scripts that are stored in the Blockchain development and have a stand-out location so they can be tracked and verified. A method for distributing a fair exchange while preventing party coordination in a decentralized way is provided by smart contracts. The ability to prepare reports independently of a real representative or legal representation eliminates time and money-related hassles, while enabling a more effective exchange of goods and services.

It can provide a more secure, straightforward and traceable supporting framework for the exchange of health data. The innovation can interface multiple data management systems working in storehouses and give what could be an associated and interoperable electronic well-being record framework. There are several steps involved in how healthcare data can be placed on the Blockchain and accessed seamlessly by patients and medical services suppliers:

1) The medical specialist treats the patient and stores the patient report with tests, prescriptions, and significant notes on their current well-being information framework. Then, the information fields relegated to the patient's public ID are diverted to the Blockchain through APIs. Here, an exchange is created.

2) Every exchange on the Blockchain is checked and given a one-of-a-kind character (public key) that is placed on the Blockchain.

3) Medical specialists and healthcare associations can produce an inquiry through APIs and use the patient's public key to recover the scrambled patient information.

4) Patients can approve the specialist or the medical care establishment by sharing the confidential key (which behaves like a secret word) to decode their information. Subsequently, the information remains scrambled for those without the confidential key.

From 2009 to 2017, there were more than 176 million healthcare record breaches. The security systems associated with Blockchain technology can help to better safeguard health data. Each individual has a public identifier or key and a confidential key that can be opened exclusively during the vital period. Also, hacking would be restricted by the need to track each client separately to obtain private data. Along these lines, Blockchains can provide a permanent review trail of health data.

11.4. Merging of Blockchain with artificial intelligence in healthcare

Blockchain combined with high-level data analytics and AI could be used to remove counterfeit medicines from the store network and achieve more noteworthy efficiencies. Producers, warehouses, transportation and coordinated operation organizations will be incorporated into the clinic or drugstore. Every bundle of medicine can be tracked on the Blockchain. The client can use the portable application to check whether a medication can be certified, which offers critical benefits. Counterfeit medicines do not enter the drugstore network. Simulated intelligence and data analytics make conveyance frameworks more effective. It will also help forestall cost contortions through the productive circulation of medicines. Automated administrative detailing and working with programmed installments across the production network will be permitted. AI and Blockchain innovation can work together on the nature of care in healthcare frameworks, reducing the cost of clinical business, and therefore the medical sector will turn out to be more open and reasonable. Blockchain empowers encoded data that AI needs. Blockchain innovation makes it feasible to decide the rationale associated with an algorithmically independent direction.

11.5. Drawbacks of using Blockchain in the healthcare industry

Blockchain cannot go in reverse as the data is invariable. Data permanence has always been the potentially most noteworthy downside of Blockchain. Various structures benefit from this, including the store network, monetary frameworks and so on. However, if we perceive how associations work, we need to appreciate that this changelessness should be accessible, expecting that the center points are flowing in the association. This means that a Blockchain association can be compelled by a component if it has half or a more prominent measure of hubs, which makes it vulnerable.

Gambles connected with Blockchain consolidate jurisdictional hardships, crypto assets, security and data insurance, twofold spending and distributed denial-of-service (DDoS) attacks. Some dangers have been recognized and defeated in similar imaginative leaps in the recent past, including the commercialization of the Internet and cloud handling. Fundamental ventures see all perils natural in Blockchain systems, including having the choice to recognize who is mindful and genuinely able. Blockchain is similarly helpless against some expansive programming shortcomings that can result in pernicious assaults. These noxious assaults can then be used to work with different offences such as wholesale fraud and data exfiltration (Xu 2016).

Finishing and managing Blockchain projects that are poorly designed and implemented subsequently requires a lot of well-established data on the relationship to go through the entire process. Right on time in 2019, Deloitte conducted a global Blockchain survey that identified a lack of understanding of Blockchain innovation as an important snag in embracing this innovation (Griggs 2018). The requirement to select multiple professionals in the field is also a major problem, adding another point to the drawbacks of Blockchain. Likewise, the professionals currently involved also need to be made proficient in the use of this technology and ensure that the managerial group can fully understand and accept the intricacies and consequences of a Blockchain-controlled business. If done properly and understanding all the needs and drawbacks, it can help change our business cycles to use Blockchain. Furthermore, Blockchain organizers and experts are more anxious to find more and as such will cost more, corresponding to standard designers based on their regular market level.

11.6. Conclusion and future scope

All things considered, the development of Blockchain has various applications that have serious consequences for the difficulties faced by the healthcare business. The most grounded capacity of Blockchain improvement is the future research applications, namely accessibility, security, decentralized nature, trustworthiness and confirmation standards because of the general record and block-related foundation.

Research is expected on Blockchain-related attacks and issues, such as block-keeping attacks and Blockchain mining impulses. In order to improve the facilities provided to patients and medical professionals, research plays a vital role in Blockchain implementation in healthcare. Adaptability is an immense problem as the medical sector is still a growing industry in terms of technological advancement. Blockchain use cases will prove decidedly more effective to run with the number of individuals or patients in the design increments. Further evaluation should be undertaken along with authentic global datasets that are open source to permit different specialists to take a look at the results and disseminate disclosures. Various appraisals approach the attestation of thought, and we need to explore the expected open entrances from medical affiliations and analysts together, to use actual medical data to assess the proposed structures (e.g. flexibility, security, execution, and other fundamental properties such as affirmation saving).

11.7. References

Ahram, T., Sargolzaei, A., Sargolzaei, S., Daniels, J., Amaba, B. (2017). Blockchain technology innovations. *2017 IEEE Technology & Engineering Management Conference (TEMSCON)*, 137–141.

Anjum, A., Sporny, M., Sill, A. (2017). Blockchain standards for compliance and trust. *IEEE Cloud Computing*, 4(4), 84–90.

Benchoufi, M., Porcher, R., Ravaud, P. (2017). Blockchain protocols in clinical trials: Transparency and traceability of consent. *F1000Research*, 6.

Cai, Y. and Zhu, D. (2016). Fraud detections for online businesses: A perspective from blockchain technology. *Financial Innovation*, 2(1), 1–10.

Dagher, G.G., Mohler, J., Milojkovic, M., Marella, P.B. (2018). Ancile: Privacy-preserving framework for access control and interoperability of electronic health records using blockchain technology. *Sustainable Cities and Society*, 39, 283–297.

Griggs, K.N., Ossipova, O., Kohlios, C.P., Baccarini, A.N., Howson, E.A., Hayajneh, T. (2018). Healthcare Blockchain system using smart contracts for secure automated remote patient monitoring. *Journal of Medical Systems*, 42(7), 1–7.

Kiyomoto, S., Rahman, M.S., Basu, A. (2017). On blockchain-based anonymized dataset distribution platform. *2017 IEEE 15th International Conference on Software Engineering Research, Management and Applications (SERA)*, 85–92.

Mamun, Q. (2022). Blockchain technology in the future of healthcare. *Smart Health*, 23, 100223.

Mettler, M. (2016). Blockchain technology in healthcare: The revolution starts here. *IEEE 18th International Conference on E-health Networking, Applications and Services (Healthcom)*, 1–3.

Pouraghily, A. and Wolf, T. (2019). A lightweight payment verification protocol for blockchain transactions on IoT devices. *2019 IEEE International Conference on Computing, Networking and Communications (ICNC)*, 617–623.

Sullivan, C. and Burger, E. (2017). E-residency and blockchain. *Computer Law & Security Review*, 33(4), 470–481.

Xu, J.J. (2016). Are blockchains immune to all malicious attacks? *Financial Innovation*, 2(1), 1–9.

Yue, X., Wang, H., Jin, D., Li, M., Jiang, W. (2016). Healthcare data gateways: Found healthcare intelligence on the blockchain with novel privacy risk control. *Journal of Medical Systems*, 40(10), 1–8.

List of Authors

Jyoti AHLAWAT
ECE Department
SGT University
Gurugram
Haryana
India

ALIND
Department of Virtualization
School of Computer Science
University of Petroleum and Energy Studies (UPES)
Dehradun
Uttarakhand
India

V. ANITHA
Kakatiya University
Warangal
Telangana
India

Leena ARYA
ECE Department
ITS Engineering College
Greater Noida
Uttar Pradesh
India

Manish Mohan BARAL
Department of Operations
GITAM School of Business
GITAM (Deemed to be University)
Visakhapatnam
Andhra Pradesh
India

Abhishek BHATTACHARYA
Co-founder
Whrrl
Kolkata
West Bengal
India

Prasenjit CHATTERJEE
MCKV Institute of Engineering
Liluah
West Bengal
India

Venkataiah CHITTIPAKA
School of Management Studies
Indira Gandhi National Open University
Delhi
India

Tanupriya CHOUDHURY
School of Computer Science
University of Petroleum and
Energy Studies (UPES)
Dehradun
Uttarakhand
India

Arepalli Peda GOPI
Vignan's Nirula Institute of
Technology & Science for Women
Guntur
Andhra Pradesh
India

Avita KATAL
School of Computer Science
University of Petroleum and
Energy Studies (UPES)
Dehradun
Uttarakhand
India

Abhirup KHANNA
School of Computer Science
University of Petroleum and
Energy Studies (UPES)
Dehradun
Uttarakhand
India

Praveen KUMAR
Amity University
Tashkent
Uzbekistan

Hussain Falih MAHDI
Department of Computer and
Software Engineering
University of Diyala
Baquba
Iraq

Neha MEHTA
Consultant (Engineering)
CSVTU
Bhilai
Chhattisgarh
India

Subhodeep MUKHERJEE
Department of Operations
GITAM School of Business
GITAM (Deemed to be University)
Visakhapatnam
Andhra Pradesh
India

V. Lakshman NARAYANA
Vignan's Nirula Institute of
Technology & Science for Women
Guntur
Andhra Pradesh
India

Dakshita NEGI
University of Petroleum and
Energy Studies (UPES)
Dehradun
Uttarakhand
India

Nisha PAL
CSED
Motilal Nehru National Institute
of Technology Allahabad
Prayagraj
Uttar Pradesh
India

R.S.M. Lakshmi PATIBANDLA
Vignan's Foundation for Science
Technology, and Research
Vadlamudi
Andhra Pradesh
India

P. PRAVEEN
SR University
Warangal
Telangana
India

B. RAMA
Kakatiya University
Warangal
Telangana
India

B. Tarakeswara RAO
Kallam Haranadhareddy Institute of Technology
Guntur
Andhra Pradesh
India

Saurabh RAWAT
Graphic Era University
Dehradun
Uttarakhand
India

Jatin SETHI
BNY Mellon Technology
Pune
Maharashtra
India

Vitesh SETHI
University of Petroleum and Energy Studies (UPES)
Dehradun
Uttarakhand
India

Anushree SHAH
University of Petroleum and Energy Studies (UPES)
Dehradun
Uttarakhand
India

Mohammed Ali SHAIK
SR University
Warangal
Telangana
India

Bhumika SHARMA
University of Petroleum and Energy Studies (UPES)
Dehradun
Uttarakhand
India

Roohi SILLE
University of Petroleum and Energy Studies (UPES)
Dehradun
Uttarakhand
India

Teoh Teik TOE
Nanyang Technological University
Singapore

Jung-Sup UM
Department of Geography
College of Social Sciences
Kyungpook National University
Buk-Gu
Daegu
South Korea

Dharmendra Kumar YADAV
CSED
Motilal Nehru National Institute of Technology Allahabad
Prayagraj
Uttar Pradesh
India

Index

P, S, T

Other titles from

iSTE

in

Computer Engineering

2022

HOMÈS Bernard
Advanced Testing of Systems-of-Systems 1: Theoretical Aspects
Advanced Testing of Systems-of-Systems 2: Practical Aspects

MEHTA Shikha, TIWARI Sanju, SIARRY Patrick, JABBAR M.A.
Tools, Languages, Methodologies for Representing Semantics on the Web of Things

SIDHOM Sahbi, KADDOUR Amira
Systems and Uses of Digital Sciences for Knowledge Organization (Digital Tools and Uses Set – Volume 9)

ZAIDOUN Ameur Salem
Computer Science Security: Concepts and Tools

2021

DELHAYE Jean-Loic
Inside the World of Computing: Technologies, Uses, Challenges

DUVAUT Patrick, DALLOZ Xavier, MENGA David, KOEHL François, CHRIQUI Vidal, BRILL Joerg
Internet of Augmented Me, I.AM: Empowering Innovation for a New Sustainable Future

HARDIN Thérèse, JAUME Mathieu, PESSAUX François,
VIGUIÉ DONZEAU-GOUGE Véronique
Concepts and Semantics of Programming Languages 1: A Semantical Approach with OCaml and Python
Concepts and Semantics of Programming Languages 2: Modular and Object-oriented Constructs with OCaml, Python, C++, Ada and Java

MKADMI Abderrazak
Archives in The Digital Age: Preservation and the Right to be Forgotten
(Digital Tools and Uses Set – Volume 8)

TOKLU Yusuf Cengiz, BEKDAS Gebrail, NIGDELI Sinan Melih
Metaheuristics for Structural Design and Analysis
(Optimization Heuristics Set – Volume 3)

2020

DARCHE Philippe
Microprocessor 1: Prolegomena – Calculation and Storage Functions – Models of Computation and Computer Architecture
Microprocessor 2: Core Concepts – Communication in a Digital System
Microprocessor 3: Core Concepts – Hardware Aspects
Microprocessor 4: Core Concepts – Software Aspects
Microprocessor 5: Software and Hardware Aspects of Development, Debugging and Testing – The Microcomputer

LAFFLY Dominique
TORUS 1 – Toward an Open Resource Using Services: Cloud Computing for Environmental Data
TORUS 2 – Toward an Open Resource Using Services: Cloud Computing for Environmental Data
TORUS 3 – Toward an Open Resource Using Services: Cloud Computing for Environmental Data

LAURENT Anne, LAURENT Dominique, MADERA Cédrine
Data Lakes
(Databases and Big Data Set – Volume 2)

OULHADJ Hamouche, DAACHI Boubaker, MENASRI Riad
Metaheuristics for Robotics
(Optimization Heuristics Set – Volume 2)

SADIQUI Ali
Computer Network Security

VENTRE Daniel
Artificial Intelligence, Cybersecurity and Cyber Defense

2019

BESBES Walid, DHOUIB Diala, WASSAN Niaz, MARREKCHI Emna
Solving Transport Problems: Towards Green Logistics

CLERC Maurice
Iterative Optimizers: Difficulty Measures and Benchmarks

GHLALA Riadh
Analytic SQL in SQL Server 2014/2016

TOUNSI Wiem
Cyber-Vigilance and Digital Trust: Cyber Security in the Era of Cloud Computing and IoT

2018

ANDRO Mathieu
Digital Libraries and Crowdsourcing
(Digital Tools and Uses Set – Volume 5)

ARNALDI Bruno, GUITTON Pascal, MOREAU Guillaume
Virtual Reality and Augmented Reality: Myths and Realities

BERTHIER Thierry, TEBOUL Bruno
From Digital Traces to Algorithmic Projections

CARDON Alain
Beyond Artificial Intelligence: From Human Consciousness to Artificial Consciousness

HOMAYOUNI S. Mahdi, FONTES Dalila B.M.M.
Metaheuristics for Maritime Operations
(Optimization Heuristics Set – Volume 1)

JEANSOULIN Robert
JavaScript and Open Data

PIVERT Olivier
NoSQL Data Models: Trends and Challenges
(Databases and Big Data Set – Volume 1)

SEDKAOUI Soraya
Data Analytics and Big Data

SALEH Imad, AMMI Mehdi, SZONIECKY Samuel
Challenges of the Internet of Things: Technology, Use, Ethics
(Digital Tools and Uses Set – Volume 7)

SZONIECKY Samuel
Ecosystems Knowledge: Modeling and Analysis Method for Information and Communication
(Digital Tools and Uses Set – Volume 6)

2017

BENMAMMAR Badr
Concurrent, Real-Time and Distributed Programming in Java

HÉLIODORE Frédéric, NAKIB Amir, ISMAIL Boussaad, OUCHRAA Salma, SCHMITT Laurent
Metaheuristics for Intelligent Electrical Networks
(Metaheuristics Set – Volume 10)

MA Haiping, SIMON Dan
Evolutionary Computation with Biogeography-based Optimization
(Metaheuristics Set – Volume 8)

PÉTROWSKI Alain, BEN-HAMIDA Sana
Evolutionary Algorithms
(Metaheuristics Set – Volume 9)

PAI G A Vijayalakshmi
Metaheuristics for Portfolio Optimization
(Metaheuristics Set – Volume 11)

2016

BLUM Christian, FESTA Paola
Metaheuristics for String Problems in Bio-informatics
(Metaheuristics Set – Volume 6)

DEROUSSI Laurent
Metaheuristics for Logistics
(Metaheuristics Set – Volume 4)

DHAENENS Clarisse and JOURDAN Laetitia
Metaheuristics for Big Data
(Metaheuristics Set – Volume 5)

LABADIE Nacima, PRINS Christian, PRODHON Caroline
Metaheuristics for Vehicle Routing Problems
(Metaheuristics Set – Volume 3)

LEROY Laure
Eyestrain Reduction in Stereoscopy

LUTTON Evelyne, PERROT Nathalie, TONDA Albert
Evolutionary Algorithms for Food Science and Technology
(Metaheuristics Set – Volume 7)

MAGOULÈS Frédéric, ZHAO Hai-Xiang
Data Mining and Machine Learning in Building Energy Analysis

RIGO Michel
Advanced Graph Theory and Combinatorics

2015

BARBIER Franck, RECOUSSINE Jean-Luc
COBOL Software Modernization: From Principles to Implementation with the BLU AGE® Method

CHEN Ken
Performance Evaluation by Simulation and Analysis with Applications to Computer Networks

CLERC Maurice
Guided Randomness in Optimization
(Metaheuristics Set – Volume 1)

DURAND Nicolas, GIANAZZA David, GOTTELAND Jean-Baptiste, ALLIOT Jean-Marc
Metaheuristics for Air Traffic Management
(Metaheuristics Set – Volume 2)

MAGOULÈS Frédéric, ROUX François-Xavier, HOUZEAUX Guillaume
Parallel Scientific Computing

MUNEESAWANG Paisarn, YAMMEN Suchart
Visual Inspection Technology in the Hard Disk Drive Industry

2014

BOULANGER Jean-Louis
Formal Methods Applied to Industrial Complex Systems

BOULANGER Jean-Louis
Formal Methods Applied to Complex Systems:Implementation of the B Method

GARDI Frédéric, BENOIST Thierry, DARLAY Julien, ESTELLON Bertrand, MEGEL Romain
Mathematical Programming Solver based on Local Search

KRICHEN Saoussen, CHAOUACHI Jouhaina
Graph-related Optimization and Decision Support Systems

LARRIEU Nicolas, VARET Antoine
Rapid Prototyping of Software for Avionics Systems: Model-oriented Approaches for Complex Systems Certification

OUSSALAH Mourad Chabane
Software Architecture 1
Software Architecture 2

PASCHOS Vangelis Th
Combinatorial Optimization – 3-volume series, 2nd Edition
Concepts of Combinatorial Optimization – Volume 1, 2nd Edition
Problems and New Approaches – Volume 2, 2nd Edition
Applications of Combinatorial Optimization – Volume 3, 2nd Edition

QUESNEL Flavien
Scheduling of Large-scale Virtualized Infrastructures: Toward Cooperative Management

RIGO Michel
Formal Languages, Automata and Numeration Systems 1: Introduction to Combinatorics on Words
Formal Languages, Automata and Numeration Systems 2: Applications to Recognizability and Decidability

SAINT-DIZIER Patrick
Musical Rhetoric: Foundations and Annotation Schemes

TOUATI Sid, DE DINECHIN Benoit
Advanced Backend Optimization

2013

ANDRÉ Etienne, SOULAT Romain
The Inverse Method: Parametric Verification of Real-time Embedded Systems

BOULANGER Jean-Louis
Safety Management for Software-based Equipment

DELAHAYE Daniel, PUECHMOREL Stéphane
Modeling and Optimization of Air Traffic

FRANCOPOULO Gil
LMF — Lexical Markup Framework

GHÉDIRA Khaled
Constraint Satisfaction Problems

ROCHANGE Christine, UHRIG Sascha, SAINRAT Pascal
Time-Predictable Architectures

WAHBI Mohamed
Algorithms and Ordering Heuristics for Distributed Constraint Satisfaction Problems

ZELM Martin *et al.*
Enterprise Interoperability

2012

ARBOLEDA Hugo, ROYER Jean-Claude
Model-Driven and Software Product Line Engineering

BLANCHET Gérard, DUPOUY Bertrand
Computer Architecture

BOULANGER Jean-Louis
Industrial Use of Formal Methods: Formal Verification

BOULANGER Jean-Louis
Formal Method: Industrial Use from Model to the Code

CALVARY Gaëlle, DELOT Thierry, SÈDES Florence, TIGLI Jean-Yves
Computer Science and Ambient Intelligence

MAHOUT Vincent
Assembly Language Programming: ARM Cortex-M3 2.0: Organization, Innovation and Territory

MARLET Renaud
Program Specialization

SOTO Maria, SEVAUX Marc, ROSSI André, LAURENT Johann
Memory Allocation Problems in Embedded Systems: Optimization Methods

2011

BICHOT Charles-Edmond, SIARRY Patrick
Graph Partitioning

BOULANGER Jean-Louis
Static Analysis of Software: The Abstract Interpretation

CAFERRA Ricardo
Logic for Computer Science and Artificial Intelligence

HOMÈS Bernard
Fundamentals of Software Testing

KORDON Fabrice, HADDAD Serge, PAUTET Laurent, PETRUCCI Laure
Distributed Systems: Design and Algorithms

KORDON Fabrice, HADDAD Serge, PAUTET Laurent, PETRUCCI Laure
Models and Analysis in Distributed Systems

LORCA Xavier
Tree-based Graph Partitioning Constraint

TRUCHET Charlotte, ASSAYAG Gerard
Constraint Programming in Music

VICAT-BLANC PRIMET Pascale *et al.*
Computing Networks: From Cluster to Cloud Computing

2010

AUDIBERT Pierre
Mathematics for Informatics and Computer Science

BABAU Jean-Philippe *et al.*
Model Driven Engineering for Distributed Real-Time Embedded Systems

BOULANGER Jean-Louis
Safety of Computer Architectures

MONMARCHE Nicolas *et al.*
Artificial Ants

PANETTO Hervé, BOUDJLIDA Nacer
Interoperability for Enterprise Software and Applications 2010

SIGAUD Olivier *et al.*
Markov Decision Processes in Artificial Intelligence

SOLNON Christine
Ant Colony Optimization and Constraint Programming

AUBRUN Christophe, SIMON Daniel, SONG Ye-Qiong *et al.*
Co-design Approaches for Dependable Networked Control Systems

2009

FOURNIER Jean-Claude
Graph Theory and Applications

GUEDON Jeanpierre
The Mojette Transform / Theory and Applications

JARD Claude, ROUX Olivier
Communicating Embedded Systems / Software and Design

LECOUTRE Christophe
Constraint Networks / Targeting Simplicity for Techniques and Algorithms

2008

BANÂTRE Michel, MARRÓN Pedro José, OLLERO Hannibal, WOLITZ Adam
Cooperating Embedded Systems and Wireless Sensor Networks

MERZ Stephan, NAVET Nicolas
Modeling and Verification of Real-time Systems

PASCHOS Vangelis Th
Combinatorial Optimization and Theoretical Computer Science: Interfaces and Perspectives

WALDNER Jean-Baptiste
Nanocomputers and Swarm Intelligence

2007

BENHAMOU Frédéric, JUSSIEN Narendra, O'SULLIVAN Barry
Trends in Constraint Programming

JUSSIEN Narendra
A TO Z OF SUDOKU

2006

BABAU Jean-Philippe *et al.*
From MDD Concepts to Experiments and Illustrations – DRES 2006

HABRIAS Henri, FRAPPIER Marc
Software Specification Methods

MURAT Cecile, PASCHOS Vangelis Th
Probabilistic Combinatorial Optimization on Graphs

PANETTO Hervé, BOUDJLIDA Nacer
Interoperability for Enterprise Software and Applications 2006 / IFAC-IFIP I-ESA'2006

2005

GÉRARD Sébastien *et al.*
Model Driven Engineering for Distributed Real Time Embedded Systems

PANETTO Hervé
Interoperability of Enterprise Software and Applications 2005